Mark Wallington is the author of four previous books, two of which – *Five Hundred Mile Walkies* and *Boogie up the River* – feature Boogie. He also writes for TV and radio. He has recently moved to live in Derbyshire, near the start of the Pennine Way.

PENNINE WALKIES

Mark Wallington

ARROW

Published in the United Kingdom in 1997 by
Arrow Books

5 7 9 10 8 6 4

First published in the United Kingdom in 1996 by Hutchinson

Arrow Books Limited
Random House UK Ltd
20 Vauxhall Bridge Road, London SW1V 2SA

Random House Australia (Pty) Limited
20 Alfred Street, Milsons Point, Sydney,
New South Wales 2061, Australia

Random House New Zealand Limited
18 Poland Road, Glenfield,
Auckland 10, New Zealand

Random House(Pty) Limited
Endulini, 5a Jubilee Road, Parktown 2193, South Africa

The Random House Group Limited Reg. No. 954009

www.randomhouse.co.uk

A CIP catalogue record for this book is available from the
British Library

Papers used by Random House
are natural, recyclable products made from wood grown in
sustainable forests. The manufacturing processes conform to
the environmental regulations of the country of origin

Printed and bound in United Kingdom by
Bookmarque Ltd, Croydon, Surrey

ISBN 0 09 9661411

For Francis and Daniel

Contents

1. 'I'm not going on holiday. I'm walking the Pennine Way'

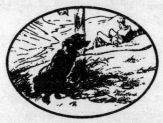

I walked my five-year-old boy to school that morning. He carried a backpack with a packet of crisps inside. I carried one with a compass, map, waterproofs, survival bag and 3 kilos of complete dog food.

Next to us walked Boogie the dog, carrying nothing, as usual.

Francis said: 'Why can't we go in the car?'

Boogie grunted in agreement.

'Because I want to walk today,' I told him.

'I hate walking,' muttered Francis.

'No you don't. Walking is good for you; walking invigorates you; walking relaxes you, clears the mind, feeds the spirit.'

'I hate walking,' muttered Francis.

'Walking is fun!'

My eyes were on the bulk of Kinder Scout rising vertically ahead of us, a camouflage-coloured cliff, low cloud hanging over it like a migraine. It looked anything but fun.

'Can I eat my crisps?' asked Francis.

'No. They're for break.'

I had some crisps for my break too, and an apple and some sandwiches. Suddenly the idea of sitting down right here outside the church and eating the lot at 8.45 A.M. was very attractive.

'It's starting to rain,' said Francis.

'It's not starting to rain.'

I sensed a note of desperation in my voice. It wasn't starting to rain . . . was it?

I said: 'Now, you remember what I've been telling you, about me going away for a while.'

'No.'

'I've been telling you for weeks now!'

'I want to be called Jason. Will you call me Jason?'

'I've been telling you that I'm going. . . .'

'. . . . to walk the Pennine Way.'

Beside me I felt Boogie tense.

'That's right. . . .'

'With Boogie. . . .' said Francis

Then I felt his lead stiffen in shock.

'That's right,' I said. 'I'll be gone a couple of weeks or so.'

'How far is the Pennine Way?' asked Francis, suddenly more serious.

'Oh . . . not far.'

'How far?'

'About 276 miles.'

A little howl came from Boogie. I felt his heels begin to drag along the tarmac.

'I can count to a thousand,' said Francis

'I know you can.'

'One two three four five. . . .'

'I want you to look after mummy and your little brother while I'm gone.'

'. . . .six seven eight nine ten eleven.'

'Don't count to a thousand now.'

'Why are cheese and onion crisps blue?'

'You mean why are the packets blue?'

'Yes. And why are salt and vinegar green?'

'It's because . . . well. . . .'

'You don't know, do you?'

'No.'

'It is raining,' said Francis.

'It's not raining.'

'Where is the Pennine Way?'

'Up there,' and I pointed up to where Kinder Scout was looming in and out of the mist. 'Up there . . . somewhere.'

We reached the school and the sign on the pub that says: Official Start of the Pennine Way.

'Why are you walking the Pennine Way?'

'Because . . . because Boogie needs a good walk.'

Boogie had cornered the postwoman now, paws wrapped round her leg, a look that said: do something! I'm being kidnapped.

I said to Francis, 'I'm going to miss you.'

And he said to me, 'I'm going to miss Boogie.'

I hugged him. 'I want to be called Jason,' he said.

'All right. Bye Jason.' I hugged him again and he wriggled loose and ran inside the school. Boogie tried to sneak in after him. I pulled him back and he gave me his 'I'd rather be anywhere else in the whole world than here now with you' expression.

Past the pub, through the hole in the wall, over the river and then there was the sign in four languages I'd passed many times before but never bothered to read:

> *Kamperen op de heide ist niet toegestaan.*
> *Defense de camper dans la lande.*
> *Zelten in der heide ist verboten.*
> *Camping on the moor is forbidden.*

And I thought: starting the Pennine Way is like crossing a border. Beyond here is another country.

I walked backwards for a while, watching the village get smaller. Then the school disappeared in trees and I turned round to face Kinder Scout, feeling guilty about having nothing to do all day except walk, feeling like I was playing truant.

What do you do when a legendary journey starts at the bottom of your garden? We'd moved from London to a house in the Edale valley, and there it was, the Pennine Way, the mother of all our trails, curving away up the hillside every time I drew back the curtains, waving at me every time I opened the front door. I didn't particularly want to walk it, but I couldn't get over just how convenient it was.

I still didn't want to walk it at Christmas when every present I got seemed to be connected to the path. Every book I unwrapped was a guide; every piece of clothing was thermal. I sat in a sweat with OS maps and followed the green dotted line as it ran ever north over high ground, out of Derbyshire's Dark Peak, through Brontë Country and into the Yorkshire Dales: on into Durham along the banks of the Upper Tees; up and over the roof of England into Northumberland; then across Hadrian's Wall and on through the great border forests to the final challenge of the Cheviots, and I thought: I don't want to walk that!

The problem with the Pennine Way is it has such a grim reputation. It's a 300 mile trudge and you come back with trenchfoot. It's over-walked and it's over-rated. It's an endurance test; people suffer pain in a variety of ways up there. And it's yesterday's path; it had its heyday in the seventies and eighties. That was what everyone said anyway. That was what I said.

But then in the New Year I met someone who sat me down and told me not to believe a word of it. 'It's a beautiful and lonely walk. It crosses windswept moors but it also follows charming rivers and dales. It passes towns and villages you won't want to leave. It goes to corners of the country you've never heard of. It's something everyone should do at some time in their life. It's a journey you'll never forget.'

And the difference between him and everyone else was that he had walked the path, and they hadn't.

As the days lengthened I began to feel the stick of inevitability prod me and push me towards the starting line. I went to the doctor with a bad back and he said: 'Poor posture! Sitting at a desk too long. Get more exercise.'

'Like walking the Pennine Way?' I said, and laughed stupidly.

'Good idea,' he nodded, and all but wrote me out a prescription. Walk this path three times a day between meals. Complete the course.

I got one of those strange chairs that help with posture. You kneel at your desk. They're so uncomfortable they make exercise seem like an attractive alternative and so you go out for a walk. Purely out of interest I climbed the first hill on the Pennine Way, just to see what was over the other side. It turned out to be another hill. So I climbed that and there was another hill and then another and another. It was addictive. I came home feeling buoyant. I'd seen no-one, and I'd found a fiver.

I began to look at the path differently, literally. I peered at it from behind bushes. I went outside on moonlight nights and looked up at the scar that the first mile has cut into the hillside and it was glowing in the dark. As spring approached I watched hikers walk past our garden carrying packs so big they looked like they were migrating. They headed into the hills with their heads down, saying nothing, as if they knew something no-one else did. One night, there was a knock on our door and there stood a middle-aged man wearing a balaclava and size twelve boots.

He looked as though he'd just escaped from somewhere. He said he was from Stoke.

'I'm looking for my friend Bob,' he mumbled.

'Sorry can't help.'

'I was meeting him off the train . . . We're going to walk the Pennine Way.'

I sat him down in the kitchen, gave him tea and biscuits and said: 'come on tell me the truth.'

'What truth?'

'Why are you really walking the Pennine Way?'

'Oh, it's something I've always wanted to do.'

'Yes yes, but really, why?'

'Er . . . the challenge.'

'Why?'

'Well, I want to . . . get back to basics. I want to, you know, find the man within. So does Bob. I want to show them at the office I can do it. To be honest, I'm not getting any younger and I want to do it now before my varicose vein gets any worse.'

That night I decided I was going to walk this path sooner or later, so why not do it sooner and get it over with. All I needed was a shove, and it came when I discovered I was in the midst of a mid-life crisis, and the Pennine Way was the only way to resolve it.

What was interesting was that it wasn't my mid-life crisis I was in the midst of. It was Boogie's.

. . . .HAS OPEN HEART SURGERY.

That was the half-a-headline in a newspaper spread over the floor; Boogie was lying over the other half.

It was a few months before we left. I was slouched in an armchair, eating a fried egg sandwich and watching a soccer international. Boogie was lying on the hearth rug, chin on the remote control, belly resting on the newspaper, one eye on the football, the other on my sandwich.

I tugged at the paper. I wanted to know who had had open heart surgery. Boris Yeltsin perhaps? Or Pavarotti, or maybe the Pope? It must have been someone unlikely, someone who shouldn't be having heart surgery. Maybe it was someone younger? Someone my age perhaps, someone like Mike Oldfield or Graham Gooch. I checked my heart rate and banished all thoughts of another fried egg sandwich.

. . . .HAS OPEN HEART SURGERY. I pulled the paper from under Boogie and it tore. I was left clutching Today's Birthdays. Joan Armatrading singer 45 – she was never 45! Must be a mistake. Billy Bremner former Scottish football captain 53 – Billy Bremner, was he really that old? Dr Lionel Kopelowitz, former president Board of Deputies of British Jews 69. Ha! I was 27 years younger than him. At 42 I was younger than everyone on the page in fact, apart from Kenneth Branagh who was 35. But he was exceptional, everyone said that. I shouldn't worry about being older than him. He was one of those workaholics. Anyone could be that successful at 35 if they tried as hard as he did. It was probably Kenneth Branagh who had had the open heart surgery.

I tugged the paper once more. Boogie gave me his 'I'm not budging unless you give me a bite of your sandwich' face.

I threw him a crust – just out of his reach. He sighed, which did he want more: a biscuit, or a good drool over the sight of a biscuit? With great effort he levered his body forward and I pulled out the newspaper.

DOG HAS OPEN HEART SURGERY.

That's what it said. A dog had had a bypass operation and was making good progress. 'Makes you think, doesn't it, Boogie?' I said. But it didn't make him think. It made him mindlessly scratch his ear with his back foot, a manoeuvre that has always impressed me.

DOG HAS OPEN HEART SURGERY.

It was a pedigree of course, a labrador, probably had it
done on BUPA. Dogs like Boogie, whose pedigree went
back as far as the knee-trembler his mother had behind
the Finsbury Park bus garage six years ago, would have to
wait 12 months for something similar on the NHS.

I looked at him lying there, a hairy lump of inertia.
You could almost hear his arteries hardening. He perked
up briefly as England had a goal disallowed and a dog
trotted onto the pitch and gave all the stewards a run.
They couldn't catch him and the crowd cheered him
on. Boogie watched wistfully, the look of a dog who
knows he is too old and unfit now ever to interrupt play
for England.

It wasn't always like this of course. It's hard to believe
but Boogie was a puppy once, a slip of a thing, a streamlined
hound standing on a hilltop with the poise of a trig point; a
beach bum running up and down the sands with a container
of toxic waste in his mouth; a street-wise mutt with a
savvy inherited from a long line of urban hybrids, half-dog
half-double decker.

But now he's reached middle age and moved to the
country. Now he spends his days lying outside the back
door wondering if he's about to be replaced by a younger
dog, and his evenings spread-eagled by the fire like a
mongrelskin rug. The only time his heart rate goes
up is when he's watching the greyhound racing on
Sportsnight.

Half-time, and an advert for complete dog food came
on. A creature that looked like a canine Tom Cruise
bounded across the screen, all sparkling teeth and exquisite
bone structure. Boogie tucked his head under his armpit,
unable to be reminded of the dog he once used to be. The
germ of an idea entered my head. I dragged him up the
stairs and put him on the scales. Three and a half stone

he weighed. But for dogs you multiplied by seven didn't you? That made him twenty four and half stone.

I looked into his eyes, cloudy and brown; he didn't have bags under them so much as dustbin liners. And look at those grey hairs on his belly, and his sagging bum and his droopy jowl, and those tramlines on his brow. I held him up in front of the mirror and said: 'Boogie, let's face it, you've been mugged by time. You're going through what every male goes through in middle age. You feel insecure about your future. You feel threatened by younger dogs. You're concerned about your appearance and whether bitches still find you attractive. You're depressed because suddenly your youth is waving at you from some distant hill and because you've no personal pension scheme. You need to be convinced you can still compete. I bet you're even worried about your prostate. You need a tonic, Boogie, a panacea!'

I opened the front door and there was the local panacea, curving away up the hillside, glowing in the dark.

I sat on the front step and wondered how I could break the news to him that his time had come to walk the Pennine Way. 'Boogie,' I said. 'How would you like to rediscover your lost youth? How would you like to look that dog in the complete dog food advert?'

And he belched and went back inside as the second half started, and I was left there wondering if the Pennine Way was visible from space.

'I'm just going for a walk with the dog and I may be some time.'

No no, that wouldn't work. That would have been the undiplomatic way to leave. Although I have to admit I've always felt a certain affinity with that sort of escapee, the sort who say they're just going out to walk the dog or get a newspaper and that's the last anyone ever sees of them.

I mean, what happens to those people? Do they begin life with a new identity on a South Pacific Island? Do they get abducted by aliens? Do they bump their heads on lampposts and everything goes blank? Or do they just keep walking the dog? Come to think of it, what happens to all those dogs?

I imagined Catherine sitting at the kitchen table while a policeman took notes. 'Had your husband . . . shown any signs of strange behaviour recently?'

'No.'

'He didn't give any clues as to where he might be going?'

'No.'

'Did he take anything with him?'

'He did have a rucksack with a series of OS maps, some waterproofs, a whistle and a 3 kilo bag of complete dog food.'

Just a daydream. If I was really going to walk the Pennine Way the time would have to be negotiated. The way to do it I decided was to dig out that line from our child-free past, the one that went: 'we always promised ourselves that once a year we'd allow each other time to do something on our own.'

Breakfast, our house, one morning in May, 1995, and there's Mr Nonchalance with a mouthful of Fruit and Fibre saying: 'what would you say if I told you I wanted to walk the Pennine Way?'

She didn't flinch. She said, 'I'd say that's a great idea.'

'Oh. Good.'

Well that was easy.

'The kids would love it. And it would give me a break as well.'

It was never going to be that easy of course. I said: 'Oh, it's too long a walk for the kids to do.'

'Take your time, do it in the school holidays.'

'You see I was thinking of doing it with the dog.'

'The dog! Which dog?'

'Boogie.'

'You'll kill him.'

'He needs a good walk. He'll be having a bypass operation if he doesn't get some good exercise soon.'

'You're proposing to leave me for two weeks with two young children just to get the dog fit.'

'Maybe three.'

'What?'

'Weeks. Not children.'

'What are you trying to prove here?'

'I'm not trying to prove anything. The dog needs a challenge. He's at that time of life. The Pennine Way is something every dog would love to do, but he needs to do it now while he still can. He needs to do something to get some spark back in him.'

'That dog wouldn't spark if you shoved a Roman candle up. . . .'

'Don't be cruel.'

It was time for the trump card. 'Do you remember how we always promised ourselves that when we had children we'd give each other time once a year to do something on our own?'

She looked up from fixing the washing machine and said: 'Did we say that?'

'Yes.'

She was gone by the weekend, gone to France with an old friend who likes to lead her astray. I spent a week combining intensive childcare with late nights reading up on peat.

Since I'd told people I was going to walk the Pennine Way, I'd noticed a marked change in reactions. No longer did they make comments like: 'The Pennine Way? They've paved it haven't they?' Now they shook their heads and warned: 'make sure you take a survival bag.' 'What are you going to do about loneliness?' 'Hope you can use a compass.'

I wasn't sure I could use a compass, so I took a short course at the local youth hostel. Over four sessions in the classroom and out on the hills a group of us learned how to navigate using contours, how to judge distances, how it's a bad idea to unfold a map in a gale, and how it's a very bad idea to take a bearing off a sheep.

We also learnt how the weather in the Pennines can turn from sunny to Arctic in minutes. We sheltered behind rocks as sleet fell on our sandwiches. Enthusiasm was fading until our instructor dropped into the conversation that he was a test model for outdoor equipment. All interest in navigation ceased at that point, and we turned our attention to the more serious matter of what make his jacket/trousers/hat/ were, what they cost him and where did he buy them.

This was my first experience of hikers doing what they do best: discuss equipment. 'I want you to recommend a jacket with good directional breathability,' demanded an accountant from King's Lynn.

'Has your fleece got a durable water repellent elastomer?' inquired a sociology student from the University of Middlesbrough.

'What do you think of trousers with articulated knees?' asked a software salesman from Cardiff.

Equipment discussion is nothing new among outdoor enthusiasts but it's never been so complex as it is now. This is because outdoor equipment has become so scientific you need a physics qualification to buy so much as a pair of socks. Kitting yourself out for a hike like the Pennine Way used to be a case of packing a change of clothes, a cagoule, a compass and map and a first aid kit. Now you're considered a danger to yourself unless you have a 'system' with boots that have the right membrane and an anorak that possesses adequate stress resistance. And you wouldn't dare leave home without wearing an undershirt that took moisture away from the body.

'How much was your hat?' asked a hairdresser from Beckenham, pointing to the silly wedge-shaped job on the instructor's head.

'Twelve quid,' said the instructor.

And the other thing about modern equipment is that it is all outrageously expensive.

Well, I wasn't having anything to with this, I decided. I was just going to polish up my old boots and be done with it. But when I polished up my old boots, I discovered they were falling apart. I took them to be repaired and it was the first time I've been laughed at by a shoe shop assistant.

I went for a second opinion to a place that specialised in restoring hiking boots. There they didn't laugh at all. They gently said: 'I think you'd better talk to Chris.'

Chris came out from the back and studied my boots. He was a sensitive man, highly skilled in counselling hikers who have become sentimental over their footwear. He sat me down, established eye contact and said: 'Had these a while haven't you?'

'Thirteen years.'

'Covered a few miles, by the look of them.'

'I walked the South West coastal path in them.'

'There's a part of you in these boots, isn't there?'

'I suppose there is.'

'They represent the freedom and footloose lifestyle you used to lead, don't they?'

'In a way, yes.'

'How old are you now?'

'42.'

'Chuck 'em out and get a new pair.'

I ended up in an activity emporium, a labyrinthine

supermarket of outdoor equipment from all over the world
that smelled of man-made fibre and money. As I wandered
through, looking for footwear, climbers were clinging to
the climbing wall like spiders; mountaineers were standing
in a corner growing their beards and talking ropes; cavers
with pale faces were trying on wellies. I found the boot
department, and to my amazement quickly settled on a pair
that were comfortable and were a good price and I was very
happy with, but then I made the mistake of telling that to a
salesperson and he wasn't happy at all.

'Oh we don't recommend those,' he said

'Why not?'

'They're not very good. Not for walking'

'They're a walking boot, aren't they?'

'Yes, but they're more for just looking good.'

'What's wrong with looking good? I want to look
good.'

'They don't respond to stress well.'

'That's perfect. Neither do I.'

'Where are you going to use them?'

'The Pennine Way.'

'Oh we don't recommend the Pennine Way.'

I tried on ten other pairs of boots from ten parts of
the world, all named after ten different mountains I
would never climb. Eventually I managed to persuade
the salesman to sell me a pair that cost £90, and he
looked at me as if I were a cheapskate. 'Don't say I didn't
warn you,' was written all over his face as I handed him
my credit card.

I moved on to anoraks. Here the choice was just as
mesmerising, and of course they weren't anoraks at all,
they were breathable clothing combinations, the result of
teams of scientists working in isolation in Arizona. I asked
the assistant: 'What exactly is Nikwax Analogy?'

'It works the same way that an animal's fur does,' he

said. 'Nikwax have analysed the methods mammals use to control temperature and waterproofing and have by analogy recreated the effect. It's simple really.'

I said: 'How did people ever go on long distance walks before? How did they manage?'

'No-one really knows. They must have suffered enormously and not realised it.'

I wondered what the staff in this place wore when they went out into the hills. Working in this sort of shop surely they wouldn't earn the money to pay for a set of Dryflo Active Thermal Underwear or a jacket with zonal layering. I found an assistant who was a little older than the rest, looked more wise. I asked him: 'Do you go hiking?'

'Been hiking all my life.'

'Which one of these outfits do you use, then?'

'Oh I can't afford any of these,' he laughed.

Of course he couldn't. It was just as I thought, this was the designer range they sold to mugs. The real stuff was out the back in a plain box and you just had to give a nod and wink and you could be kitted out for thirty quid.

'So what do you wear?' I asked.

'Nothing.'

'Nothing?'

'No.'

'What do you do when it rains?'

'I get wet and cold and wish I could afford a breathable jacket.'

In the end I bought an anorak and over-trousers set for twenty-five pounds that couldn't breathe and didn't have a membrane and was made in Taiwan.

Finally I arrived at the accessory counter where I discovered I needed one of everything: survival bag, mini-torch, waterproof matches, copy of *Wuthering Heights*. And some emergency rations of course. Although rations isn't really the word here. Gone are the days when you packed a bar of Kendal Mint Cake and some dried fruit. Now there are three-course dehydrated meals on offer in envelope-sized packs, and a choice that includes Madras curry, chicken with almonds and beef stroganoff. I perused the menu and ordered the *duck à l'orange*. It was a great comfort to know I could be suffering from exposure on Black Hill but would still be able to prepare a candlelight dinner.

All that remained on my list was a whistle. But I thought: why bother with a whistle? I'd have Boogie with me. He'd be like Lassie in times of trouble. If I fell and injured myself he'd charge off to the nearest mountain rescue station and raise the alarm. The team leader would look him in the eye and say: 'He's trying to tell us something. What is it, boy?' And Boogie would bark out a map reference and the team would scramble; and just as I was about to slip into a coma a helicopter would appear and there would be Boogie descending on a winch. . . .

'I'd like a whistle, please,' I asked the woman at the accessory counter, expecting to be shown The Zenith Whistle Range, whistles that would work to a depth of 300 feet and a height of 30,000, that would glow in the dark and keep moisture away from the lips when blown.

And I expected to be shown at least five models ranging from the Snowdon to the Everest, all of which were endorsed by Chris Bonington and recommended by the Mountaineering Club, and all came in a waterproof pack and had instructions on 'how to look after your new Zenith whistle'. And I expected to pay nothing less than £6.95.

But the assistant reached behind her, plonked a piece of orange plastic on the counter and said: 'there.'

'What's that?'

'A whistle.'

'What make?'

'I don't know. It's the only one there is.'

I looked at it suspiciously. 'It's a proper whistle, is it? Not a second or anything. I mean there's nothing wrong with it?'

'No.'

'How much?' If the company had a monopoly they could charge at least fifteen quid.

'60p.'

I had my money down on the counter and I was out of there before she'd rung the till, and I blew my new whistle all the way home.

I began a period of preparation. I considered camping, but Boogie is the kind of animal who is reluctant to travel anywhere unless there's satellite TV in the room and a mini-bar, and anyway there was such a variety of cheap accommodation available along the Pennine Way – hostels, bunk barns, B&Bs – I didn't see much point in taking a tent. I'd take a sleeping bag and a stove but otherwise weight would be kept to the minimum. I discarded the top to my pen. I half-emptied my tube of toothpaste.

I wore my new boots all day long. I sat at my desk in them. I watched a one-day cricket international on TV in them. I even went walking in them. I carried Daniel, my two-year-old, in a backpack up the first mile of the Pennine Way. He fell asleep as soon as I strapped him in, and since he weighed about the same amount as my pack would when fully-laden, this was perfect training.

Boogie too adopted a fitness regime. This consisted of eating a lot more and panting on the spot. He polished up his little-dog-lost look, the one designed to zap a stranger at 50 metres and coax a boiled sweet out of him. He practised jumping in the back seat of vehicles. He practised his limp. He even came out on walks with me and Daniel. His problem, though, is that he has no idea he's not as young as he used to be. He's used to walks that last the length of a commercial break, and he sprints away at the start like a young whippet then wonders why within 200 yards he's leaning against a tree coughing and frothing and feeling chest pains. I tried to convince him of the need to pace himself. He tried to convince me of his need to take the place of Daniel in the backpack.

I thought it best to take him to the vet for a check-up. We sat in the waiting room opposite a poster advert for complete dog food. There was that model dog again, pouting and posing. 'That's what you're going to look like when this walk is over,' I said to Boogie. And he sat there thinking: great! I'm going to have plastic surgery.

The vet examined him and said: 'does your dog smoke?'

'No.'

'Drink alcohol?'

'Only the occasional sweet sherry with the family at Christmas.'

'In that case a damn good walk would do him the world of good.'

I asked the vet to take a picture of us for a before-and-after shot. I'm standing there in the street outside his surgery adopting the classic poise of a Pennine Way walker, body leaning at an angle of 65 degrees into the wind. Boogie, by contrast, has the look of a confused pet, a look that says: I'm not entirely sure what's going on here but I've a feeling it might mean missing Wimbledon Fortnight.

Catherine came home with a suntan and bottle of duty free, looking years younger. For a few days I wondered if maybe there wasn't a Pennine Way equivalent I could walk in the south of France, but by this time I was dreaming of the Pennines. One night the path was a conveyor belt and walkers stepped on it to be transported effortlessly to Scotland. It was like a cruise and the deck was dotted with people playing quoits and clay pigeon shooting.

Another night a group of hikers were gathered around me looking concerned and asking me if I knew that my clothing system wasn't breathing.

A third night I was sitting by a camp fire eating complete dog food, and Boogie was next to me with a napkin tucked into his collar, eating *duck à l'orange* by candlelight. I woke and decided I needed to get going as soon a possible.

I consulted long range weather reports and tried to contact that weather guru in Thirsk who makes his predictions by observing the moles, but in the end I just picked a date a week ahead. I spent the last few days mowing the lawn very short and putting up smoke alarms all round the house, one eye always on the hills.

'I wish you'd get going,' Catherine said on the Friday.

'Monday morning you'll think differently,' I replied.

But when Monday dawned it was me who was thinking differently. I pulled back the curtains and where I normally saw the path curving away up the hill now I saw nothing, just a gloom and a thin drizzle, and when I stuck my head out of doors there was a chill air on my ears. 'Bastards,' I muttered, unsure who to blame for this but wanting to blame someone.

I woke Boogie up and packed my bag; woke Boogie up again, and ate two fried eggs. I yelled Walkies! as loud as I could in Boogie's ear and pulled my rucksack on. Eventually he stirred and followed me, grumbling, as far as the doormat where he lay down again and looked at me to say: listen, if you want me to go for a walk at this time of the morning I'm going to need drugs, all right.

Daniel said: 'Francis going to school. Mummy going to work. Daddy going on holiday.'

'I am not going on holiday. I am going to walk the Pennine Way.'

'Good luck,' Catherine said and pinned a charm to my
T-shirt. 'This is from China. I can't remember if it keeps
travellers safe or brings rain.'

I hugged her hard and walked down the garden path.
At the gate I turned, gave her one last look, and said
as affectionately as possible: 'Don't forget to put out the
dustbins on Sunday night.'

We headed up Grindsbrook. I looked back again and saw
the village rooftops reappear briefly through the trees, then
we entered the mist and the valley was gone and I felt
under sail.

Boogie lagged behind, looking very worried now.
Surely I was going to stop soon, ruffle his head and say:
'just kidding, we're going to the pub really.'

We reached the first challenge of the journey: a kissing
gate. I slipped through and expected Boogie to follow but
he just stood there. I was all for male bonding on this trip
but if he thought I was kissing him within range of Edale
he was mistaken.

Then I realised he couldn't fit round. The next ten
minutes were spent navigating this first gate of the walk.
I tried pulling him through. He tried pulling me back. I
slipped on some mud in the struggle and he eyed me with
a: 'good idea; pretend you've sprained an ankle and we can
turn back; it's not too late; I won't tell a soul.'

I said: 'You either squeeze through or sit there until you
get thinner.' He chose to sit there. In the end I picked him
up and bundled him over. 'And if you think I'm doing that
all the way to Scotland you've another think coming.'

I climbed slowly, encouraging the tops to clear, enjoying
the sound of running water everywhere. The walk up
Grindsbrook is a lovely one no matter what the weather,
and I felt pleased with myself for just being here: 'Don't
you feel better already? Can't you feel that feeling? The

one you haven't felt since . . . the last time you felt it? This walk is going to change your life!'

I looked down at Boogie and he was slouching along with an old biscuit wrapper in his mouth. I snatched it from him and pocketed it. How could anyone drop litter in such a beautiful place? I decided to pick up any rubbish I found on this path and put it in a bin.

Before I'd gone a mile my pockets were full and I had a plastic bag strapped to my pack stuffed with drink cans, orange peel and crisp packets. I scrambled up towards the ridge, grumbling about the human race and thinking: just why are cheese and onion crisps in a blue packet anyway? They should be green, surely. Cheese and onion was much more of a green colour than a blue colour. But salt and vinegar had the green packet. Odd.

I had 276 miles to think about things like that.

2. Peak Park Pie

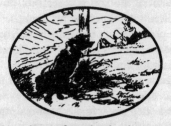

A friend of mine has a friend who knows someone who was once out on Kinder Scout when a blanket fog came down. He lost the path in visibility so bad he couldn't see his feet. He began to prod his way forward with a stick. Suddenly he could feel nothing but thin air in front of him. He thought he must be on the edge of one of the cliffs that rim the plateau, so he turned round, but then he could feel nothing behind him either. He prodded to the left – nothing; prodded to the right – nothing. He didn't dare move. He just stood on the same spot for three hours until the fog lifted, and then he discovered his stick had broken.

Kinder Scout is rich in urban mythology. It's the sort of place Japanese soldiers who still think the war is on brush shoulders with recently landed aliens and radioactive sheep. And then there's that ghost of the Pennine Way walker who perished an hour into his journey and is now doomed to roam the moors for eternity asking anyone he sees: 'where did you buy your jacket and how much was it?'

But tall stories are unnecessary here. The real thing is daunting enough. As you climb up from Edale the trail quickly narrows and reaches for the sky. Gone are the smooth, green limestone hills of the White Peak where people sit in cars and read their horoscopes in newspapers. You're heading for the Dark Peak, and a black line of broken gritstone teeth. No-one comes up Kinder Scout in search of a cream tea.

The last mile to the top is a scramble over rocks. But the urge to know what lies beyond the lip of the 2000-foot cliff draws you on. When you finally pull yourself up and peer over, your reward is to understand how the explorers Blacksland, Lawson and Wentworth felt in 1813 when, having searched for years for a way through Australia's Blue Mountains to the rich pastures they were convinced lay on the other side, they finally found a pass and emerged to look down on 5000 miles of desert.

Kinder Scout is often referred to as a desert, although this is being unfair to deserts. It's basically a high moorland plateau of gritstone, onto which time has dumped a few million lorryloads of peat, and erosion has carved a tangled network of high-sided channels known as peat groughs. It looks like the mould from which oceans are cast.

There is a designated route across but navigation is never easy. Secondary trails continually lure you off course, and the terrain is so featureless that map-reading becomes a guessing game. The temptation is to walk in the peat groughs because they have a good firm base compared to the porridge-like consistency of the moor's surface. But the problem is that their sides are too high to see over, and so you walk with no overall visibility. You just follow the channel, peering round corners, wondering where it's going to take you. This is nature's attempt at a maze and it's a good one, and if there's one thing Kinder Scout could benefit from, it's an attendant on an elevated umpire's chair, like the uniformed one they have at Hampton Court, shouting instructions from above to the lost and the crying.

Thankfully the visibility was beginning to improve as I set out on the passage across. The cloud was sliding off the moor like an eiderdown off a bed. I could see the outlines of the peat caps rolling away into the distance, and I strode off in search

of the head of the Kinder River which I knew would lead
us to Kinder Downfall, the first landmark on the journey.

I'd been up here a number of times before and had
found the riverhead without much trouble, but today felt
different; today I felt nervous. I found myself constantly
monitoring my body, expecting a part of me to malfunction
without warning. A grouse with a clown-red nose took off
like a helicopter directly in front of us and banked with a
manic screech. Boogie and I both yelped and he leapt up
into my arms only because I didn't leap into his first. We
stood there clutching each other. My heart was thumping.
Boogie's heart was thumping. Man and Dog Found Dead
on Moor in Bizarre Heart Attack Pact.

The peat was soft and dry, like walking in slippers, and
so quiet I could hear myself swallow. So where were all
these crowds of walkers when you wanted them? When it
was your first day out and you could use a friend, someone
to nod your head to and say: 'nice day for it.' Whenever
anyone had said to me: 'the Pennine Way is a motorway,'
I'd thought: suits me, I don't want to be alone up there, the
more the merrier. But the only people I saw all morning
were three hikers on the horizon. We passed like ships,
rising and falling into the peat groughs. I went down into
one and when I emerged they were gone for ever.

'I'll talk to you,' I said to Boogie. 'We're companions
after all. The idea is to keep each other company. So.
Nice day for it isn't it? Where did you get that collar from
and how much was it? Did you see that episode of Peak
Practice last night?'

His face was like: 'Why not bring the cat along instead
of me? The cat would love this. Let me run back and
get her.'

A curlew screamed overhead on low level flying
manoeuvres. I followed its flight to where the land
dipped and there I could make out the Kinder River,

a wide and sandy channel and I felt better as we stepped
down onto its dry bed. Boogie too seemed more at ease
walking on sand. He's always liked the beach ever since
he seduced a deck chair attendant's blue poodle behind
the ice cream kiosk at Broadstairs. He may well have been
recalling this memory as he turned a bend in the river and
came face to face with a doberman.

Boogie froze. The doberman circled him and licked his
lips. Boogie is by nature a pacifist, which impresses humans
but is the cause of much derision among other dogs. The
doberman looked as though he was about to flush Boogie's
head down a peat bog for fun when his owner came jogging
round the corner with a bristling moustache.

'Nice day for it!' I said eagerly.

'Lovely day for it,' he panted.

Both man and dog looked supremely fit, and it became
evident that the doberman wasn't going to snap Boogie
in two after all. Instead he was going to shame him into
submission simply by standing there and displaying his
superbly muscular physique. He thrust his perfectly formed
shoulders forward, extended his long lean rear legs. Boogie
looked like he wanted to vomit.

'Where are you heading for?'

The man was running on the spot as he replied. 'We've
come up from the Snake Inn. We'll head down to do a
circuit of Ladybower. Then back via Ringing Roger.' I'd
only asked him to be polite – 'we'll cover about thirty-
five miles today. Just a jog' – now I wished I hadn't
bothered.

'I'm walking the Pennine Way actually,' I said, although
he hadn't asked.

'Last week we ran over Bleaklow and Black Hill
in a day.'

'I think we go that route on the Pennine Way.'

'We run a hundred miles a week, me and Shah.'

'That's about what we'll cover on *The Pennine Way*.'

'Well, when you get to our age you've got to look after yourself, haven't you?'

'Exactly.'

The doberman was rippling his neck muscles now. Boogie was looking the other way, yawning.

'How old's your dog?' I asked.

'He's five.'

'Looks younger than that.'

'He's fed plenty of fibre and he's in bed by nine every night.'

No television either I bet. Now the doberman was pushing his bum out like Mr Dog Universe. Boogie decided if we were stopping he might as well lie down and have a kip.

'How old's your dog?' asked the jogger.

'Seven,' I lied. 'Well, six and a half.'

'He looks older than that.'

'He covers a hundred miles a week. In the car.'

The man was deep breathing now, and trying to touch his nose with his knee. I wanted to ask him how old he was but I was frightened he might be older than me. And anyway he looked like he was in a hurry. 'Come on, Shah,' he said. Shah did a pirouette around Boogie, and man and dog trotted off. Boogie had found a cigarette end from somewhere.

'Don't be intimidated,' I said, as we continued along the riverbed. 'It doesn't happen overnight, you know. You have to put in a bit of effort to get like that. But that's how you'll look by the time we get to Scotland. Lean and vibrant. Other dogs will admire you as you cruise past. Stop chewing that cigarette end.'

The river widened, the channel sloped and filled with rocks. There was a lot more sky and wind, and finally the land gave way to a view that was enough to jumpstart any flagging spirit. Kinder Downfall, a grand old gritstone cliff edge with a rockfall tumbling down the steep slopes. It looked like a ruin.

I sat in a cleft, out of the chilly wind, and brewed up a cup of tea. The weather mustered to the west, adding drama to the fine view down to Manchester. It wouldn't have felt right to be up here in shirt-sleeves on a warm and sunny day. These crags needed a menacing sky.

Boogie dropped a sweet wrapper at my feet and I picked it up to pocket it. But this was no ordinary piece of litter, this had Japanese writing on. It was proof that people come to Kinder Scout from all over the world to drop litter.

For this is a hallowed spot to any lover of the outdoors. It was up here one Sunday morning in 1932 that the famous Mass Trespass took place, when 400 ramblers gathered below in Hayfield and marched onto the grouse moors of Kinder Scout, to protest about the appalling lack of access that the public had to these hills and to the countryside as a whole.

This was at a time of huge recession. There were 3 million unemployed, many of them youngsters in their twenties with no money and lots of energy. To them the hills represented the only escape from the smoke of the city, and yet all this beautiful country was managed solely for the grouse shoot, and fiercely guarded by gamekeepers.

It all came to a head that Sunday as rambler met gamekeeper head on. The gamekeepers formed a defensive line on one of the ledges but the ramblers brushed them aside and reached the Downfall to rendezvous with other trespassers who had climbed by different routes. Arrests were later made and five were imprisoned but the day inevitably belonged to the ramblers. Public access gradually improved until in 1951 the Peak National Park was opened. Now you can wander anywhere you like on this moor.

It was on the back of this campaign for increased access

that the idea for the Pennine Way was born. A journalist on the *Daily Herald* named Tom Stephenson had been inspired by long distance paths in America, and in 1935 he wrote an article suggesting a trail be created that would follow the Pennine chain. The idea was enthusiastically received all the way to parliament, and although it took forty years before all the rights of way were negotiated, once the route opened its popularity was immediate. There was something peculiarly and wonderfully English about spending your holidays wading through peat bogs in the rain. Now, finding a Japanese sweet wrapper on Kinder Downfall confirmed what I had already suspected: the Pennine Way had entered the culture, it was part of the national tour. Overseas tourists had a day in Stratford, a day in Bath and a good hike over Kinder, and they'd done England.

It was shortly after midday that I encountered another Pennine Way walker. Boogie and I had followed the line of crags that border the Kinder plateau and were coming down across the hogsback of squelch known as Featherbed Moss. Now there were views of Sheffield to the east to complement those of Manchester to the west, but the tall figure striding towards us dominated all aspects.

He was obviously walking the Pennine Way. He had a big pack high on his back and his huge beard was visible from a distance. I wondered how to greet him, wondered if we'd stop and do lunch, swop Pennine Way stories. Maybe we'd swop addresses and keep in touch, send each other Christmas cards: hope to see you in '96. Maybe I'd be Godfather to his next child.

Or maybe we'd walk straight past each other as you would in a busy street, saying nothing.

Maybe he'd mug me.

The closer he got the more he looked like Clint Eastwood of the Pennines. He'd probably started out small but now after weeks on the road he was a giant. He wore shorts and gaiters. He had a tanned face, forearms and knees. In the bath he would look like something chocolate and vanilla. We slowed. We stopped. I let him have the first word:

'You come over Kinder?'

Now he reminded me of Little John standing there blocking my way, his voice was so deep it cast a shadow.

'Yep,' I said, 'Been there, done that,' and giggled.

He nodded, as if to say: that's how I was when I started, kid.

'Where have you come from?' I asked.

He'd walked the Pennine Way all right. He'd also walked across Scotland on the Southern Upland Way before that. Now he was walking home to Matlock. It was the sort of thing he did every year. His family took him to some faraway place and then left him to walk back home. He was like a clockwork dad who they wound up and let go. They just had to be ready to grab him as he passed the house or he would have kept going to Land's End.

I quizzed him on the route ahead. There was still snow on Fountains Fell, he said. I could get a great breakfast in Widdybank Farm. I was to watch out for the bull in the field past Sleightholme.

Then somehow the conversation slipped imperceptively into negative equity. One minute we were two rugged adventurers who would have drunk our own urine without a thought, the next we were two lonely souls on a grey moor discussing house prices in the Midlands. 'Makes you feel so insecure,' he said, and looked as though he was going to blow his nose on his beard

Finally he said: 'It's a good idea bringing a dog, isn't it?'

'He's good company.'

'And you can eat him if you get stuck.'

'Yes.'

Then he was gone, taking big strides and big gulps of air, heading up to the fortress-like cliffs of Kinder. I wondered if he'd started off with a dog.

The Snake Road caught me unawares. I'd imagined we would take a dive down into a valley here, lose all the height we had gained and have to climb up again to cross Bleaklow, but we reached it at the summit of its pass.

I could tell this by nothing more scientific than a glance at the completely knackered cyclist who passed us as we crossed the road. The poor man was barely moving. He had reached the top and ahead was the long descent into Glossop, but his lungs had a death rattle; his chest heaved as if seismic. If you took off twenty years for the stress he was under he was probably my age and build and I had this terrible vision of June being the month when every middle-aged man in the country gets worried and heads out on a bike or on a path or up a mountain, trying to resist time, thinking if he walks that or climbs this or swims that his bald patch will sprout and his blood pressure will simmer down and that young woman who works in the dry cleaners will give him the eye.

The cyclist tried to say something, but couldn't get the words out. 'It's all downhill now,' I said gently and wanted to pat him on the back, although such a gesture could have proved fatal. He nodded and tried again to speak but realised he needed to conserve oxygen and freewheeled away.

Boogie and I set our sights on Bleaklow, another waste-land of high moor spread thickly with peat, and with a reputation similar to Kinder for swallowing the unwary.

The names of these places don't help of course. If you're feeling uneasy on your first day out, Kinder Downfall conjures up images of locals pushing their

children off a cliff. Bleaklow inspires little but a desire
to phone the Samaritans. Just glancing at the map of
the Pennines you can see them littered with names
like Dismal Hill, Withenshaw's Depression, the Vale of
Gloom. Maybe onto the equipment list of any sensible
Pennine Way walker should go a supply of Prozac.

In fact Bleaklow, like Kinder Scout, is an unnerving
more than a treacherous landscape, with a similar silence
about it, the silence of a slumbering bear. As you walk
softly over the peat the only noise is the faint trickle of
water from every crack in the ground, and there's a sense
of being in the presence of something very powerful,
something temperamental which is being lenient with you
for no reason. I found myself walking nimbly, on tiptoe, as
if I was trying not to wake anyone, trying to pass through
unnoticed, at the same time not lose the trail.

As it is you've got to be pretty stupid to lose the trail
on Bleaklow. Navigation is much easier here than across
Kinder Scout because not only do flagstones mark a good
length of the route, at regular intervals they're actually
painted with yellow markers so that even the brighter
sheep can find their way across.

Having galvanised myself, done a map and compass
course, filled my rucksack with whistles and survival
bags and sachets of dehydrated food, and made a will
and everything, this was all very disappointing. Bleaklow
was reputed to be one of the hardest parts of the whole
hike to navigate but, as far as I could see, was just a case
of following a yellow dotted line. The only confusion was
that on my map the line was coloured green.

This made it all the more embarrassing when I did get
lost. I couldn't understand how I managed it. We'd just
reached another stile and Boogie had refused again. I'd
picked him up and thrown him over, and was muttering
to him how it was funny the way some dogs had gone up

in space rockets while others were still struggling to grasp
stiles, when it dawned on me I was no longer on my yellow
brick road. Instead I was standing in the middle of a vast
moor, the meat in a sky and peat sandwich.

I headed for a group of rocks I could see in the distance,
which could only be those marked on my map as the Hern
Stones. Or were they the Wain Stones? And anyway what
was all this stuff strewn over the ground? Lumps of twisted
metal, a trail of them.

They led to the silent and sad wreckage of an aircraft,
spread over an area of moor about fifty yards square, a
lot of wreckage from a large plane. A wing lay gently
on the peat. An engine sat connected to nothing. It was
hard to tell how old it all was, some pieces were rusted but
others still gleamed. Then I found a plaque that told the
story. The aircraft was an American Airforce Superfortress
– nickname Overexposed – that had crashed in November
1948 whilst descending through cloud, killing all thirteen
crew. They were on a routine flight and heading for base;
they probably never even saw the ground.

I heard a crunch and turned to see a man seated nearby
chewing on an apple. I hadn't seen him but he'd been there
all the time.

'It's dangerous that is,' he said. 'All them sharp bits of
metal. They should take it away.'

I suggested it had been here so long it was part of the
scenery and belonged up here, but he didn't agree.

'It's just scrap. Looks like the breaker's yard near my
house in Oldham.'

It was much more than that though. The wreckage lay
there like some memorial. A faded poppy from Remembrance Day was still tucked into one of the wings.

I wandered over to the stones, which turned out to
be the Higher Shelf Stones and were covered with very
neat and heavily carved graffiti. One set of initials was

dated 1828. The view stretched down into Glossop far below and made you realise how unlucky the crew of Overexposed had been. The plane had hit the very top of the hill, right by the trig point. There are only three summits over two thousand feet in the whole of the Peak District and Higher Shelf is one of them. Another few feet of altitude and they'd have glided over and down to Glossop.

From these rocks I was able to navigate my way north to the Hern Stones, then on to the Wain Stones which are easily identified because they have been eroded into a kiss. I walked round them looking for lips, until I was convinced that the stones weren't kissing, they were looking up each other's nose and so maybe they weren't the Wain Stones after all. I was saved when I glanced at Boogie and saw he was standing on another yellow flagstone and had found the trail again. He looked at me as if I was hopeless.

From here it was a short walk to Bleaklow Head, the desolate summit, where the landscape slips into the lunar. Even the sheep here looked hard done by. Compared to their cousins down in the Cotswolds or the South Downs this bunch were living in rural deprivation.

I stood by the trig point and surveyed the sea of muddy grey. Up above, on another level of life, I could hear a jet climbing from Manchester Airport, the drinks trolley rattling down the aisle, the passengers reading airport paperbacks, all heading for two weeks somewhere very unlike the Pennine Way. Boogie and I looked up into the cloud. Both of us would probably have paid large sums of money to be on that plane.

The noise of the aircraft engines faded and we were left to the sound of the slim breeze rustling through the even slimmer cotton grass. I said quietly: 'I promise you Boogie, no matter how bad things get on this trip, I will never eat you.'

★   ★   ★

We followed Wildboar Grain as it flowed down steeply from Bleaklow into Longdendale. I'd done nothing but walk all day and the time had flown by, but now it was five o'clock, and I could hear my children coming home and the radio on and the clatter and bang of the kitchen. I could smell burnt fish fingers and hear screams as the piano lid fell on a two-year-old's thumbs. I could see the bottle of milk falling to the floor and the cat licking it up and slashing her tongue, and the phone going and smoke coming from the toaster and a banana flying across the room and the smoke alarm screaming until someone hits it with a shoe, and I felt so glad to be out on Bleaklow.

Some sort of civilisation was emerging now. We passed a factory farm guarded by chunky rottweilers who were unhappy about something. Boogie barked back, very brave with a six foot barbed wire fence between him and them.

Then a deep valley opened out and I could see a road winding up through trees. I could see reservoirs, and we were coming down into Crowden. The sound of running water, with me all day like a background noise, disappeared and I realised how I'd taken it for granted as it was replaced by the growl of lorries on tarmac.

There was a National Park hostel in Crowden. Dogs weren't normally allowed to stay, but it was a quiet night and the warden let me in. He took one look at Boogie leaning against the drinks machine and said: 'well, he looks like a bundle of fun.'

Boogie was in no mood for sarcasm. He wanted pampering and he wanted it now. He sighed disconsolately. I translated: 'He says, can he have a gin and tonic and a hot water bottle? Please.'

We were given a little room to ourselves. I laid a blanket down on the floor for Boogie and he jumped on the bunk with a 'you're sleeping down there, are you? Suit yourself.'

I gave him his dinner and he wouldn't even stand up to eat it, just stretched his neck from the prone position. He had to swallow upwards.

'It was fun today, wasn't it?' I enthused. 'I mean, you must have enjoyed it a bit. A little bit anyway. Well it was better than sitting home watching a video.'

He gave me his 'shut up and pass the Minced Morsels' look, then licked the bowl, belched, farted and went to sleep.

The hostel was a converted row of railway cottages, built in the days when Crowden was a thriving community full of work from the local quarries and from the building of the railway and the reservoirs. In those times there was a station, a school and a local squire, but then the projects that gave the village life were completed and the population dwindled. Now the railway is closed and the empty tunnels carry electricity cables instead of trains. The valley is dominated by the trans-Pennine trunk road that groans through the night.

I had an evening meal with two men from Liverpool. One of them said to me: 'It's nice and clean here, isn't it?'

'Hygienic,' said his companion.

They introduced themselves as Tony and Doug. 'Did you come over Snake Pass today?' asked Tony.

'Yes I did.'

Doug said: 'I thought it was called Snake Pass because it was a twisty road, but that's not the reason, you know. It's because of the Snake Inn further down. And that's called the Snake Inn because it belongs to the Duke of Devonshire and his coat of arms has a snake in it.'

'Duke of Derbyshire, you mean,' said Tony.

'Duke of Devonshire,' said Doug.

'This is Derbyshire,' said Tony.

Doug sighed: 'I know this is Derbyshire, but the Duke of Devonshire owns most of it.'

''Course he doesn't.'

'Yes he does.'

'What's the Duke of Devonshire owning half of Derbyshire for?' protested Tony. 'I mean the Duke of Derbyshire is going to have something to say about that, isn't he?'

'Maybe he owns chunks of Devonshire,' I said.

'Not much point in being Duke of one county if you live in another, is there?' said Tony

Doug settled things down with an equipment question. 'Are your trousers Gore-tex?' he asked me.

'No, they're not,' I said.

'Good,' said Doug.

'He doesn't like Gore-tex,' said Tony and pulled a face.

'I'm of the opinion that Gore-tex is overrated,' said Doug.

This was a very controversial thing to say. Most walkers lie awake at night dreaming of the day they'll own a Gore-tex jacket. To say Gore-tex is over-rated is enough to provoke a letter to the editor of the *Rambler*.

A chef appeared and mumbled 'Chocolate pudding,' and left three bowls steaming on the counter. They contained something the same colour and consistency as the peat we'd walked across all day. It looked as though he'd stepped outside and cut a chunk out of the Peak Park.

The empty dining room echoed to the sound of youth hostel cutlery on youth hostel china. I didn't want to ask Tony and Doug if they were walking the Pennine Way in case they said yes and I was stuck with them for the rest of the journey. Then it struck me that they didn't want to ask me if I was walking the Pennine Way for the same reason. The tension got too much,

though. At the same time we all said: 'Are you walking
the. . . . ?'

'Sorry, after you,' I said.

'No, after you,' said Doug.

I took a breath: 'I was just wondering if you were
walking the. . . . ?'

'The . . . ?' asked Doug.

'Yes, the. . . .'

'Pennine Way?' asked Tony.

'Are you walking the Pennine Way?' I asked.

'Yes,' said Tony proudly. 'Are you?'

'No.'

'Oh.'

'Well, maybe. See how it goes.'

The chef poked his head round.

'More pudding?'

He looked so hurt that no-one was going to have any
more that I took another bowl.

'Oh well, early start,' said Doug.

'Yeah, early start,' said Tony.

And they left me alone with a mouthful of Peak
Park pie.

There didn't appear to be much to do in Crowden except
say: 'oh well, early start,' to anyone who would listen, and
then go to bed. I wandered round the hostel and read the
fire drills and the breakfast menu and looked at maps on
walls, and I was about to turn in when up on the landing I
came across a framed newspaper-clipping, and if this was to
be believed then Crowden was far from lifeless. Here was
a full page feature that claimed this little community was a
hotbed of satanism and ghostly goings-on. A reporter talked
of naked dancing in the churchyard. 'Doesn't surprise me,'
one local was quoted. 'All par for the course.'

There was also an account of Roman legions seen on

Bleaklow at night, lines of lights marching across the moors. The story caught my eye because in my family we had a wacky Uncle Jimmy who came from Manchester and once claimed he saw a Roman centurion on the Snake Pass. Everyone laughed at him when he recounted this tale. Uncle Jim was a salesman for Pickering Peas and also known for trading in tall stories. Meeting a Roman centurion on Snake Pass was the kind of thing you expected to happen to him, and you said: 'really Jim? you don't say,' and went back to reading the cereal packet. But now here, long after his death, was his vindication.

I took Boogie outside. There was a tree about thirty yards away but he wasn't going to walk that far. Instead he imagined a birch right where he was and cocked his leg on it.

I glanced up at Bleaklow. No Roman centurions abroad tonight. No lights in the sky or naked dancing either, just the sound of trucks squashing small mammals on the A645.

'Nothing improves a view like ham and eggs,' wrote Mark Twain, and how right he was. I woke to a window full of low cloud and drizzle. The hills of the previous day had a veil drawn over them. No sign of a brightening sky in any direction. Then I came down for egg and bacon and watched the cloud slowly lift and Bleaklow appear once more, looking all the more attractive to me in the knowledge that I had already come over it and wouldn't have to go anywhere near it ever again.

Although the prospect in the other direction, the one I was heading for, was no less daunting. Up there somewhere was Black Hill, the main obstacle of the day, another high lump of moorland and peat that no-one ever mentioned by name without grimacing and attaching a grisly prefix. The Unearthly Black Hill was a common one; the Unforgiving was also popular; the Morass of, was the favourite.

I dallied. The cloud may have lifted but the rain was still falling vertically. Boogie gazed at me pitifully: please tell me it's a dream, tell me we're not going out in that? Tell me we're going to stand by this radiator and read *Country Life* and eat leftover chocolate pudding all morning.

I didn't exactly feel full of vim myself. My feet ached. I had a strange pain in my hip. My shoulders were sore and my neck felt cricked. I thought: thank goodness I got myself fit before I left.

'We just need to get going,' I enthused to Boogie. 'Walk off the stiffness.' And he tried to fake an appendicitis, right there in the dining room.

I watched from the landing window as the Liverpool two set off, velcroed tightly into their waterproofs. I mooched round the hallway, reading menus I would never have to choose from. 'Still raining, huh,' I said to the warden.

''Course it's still raining,' he replied.

I bought a picnic lunch off him – took fifteen minutes to buy it off him in fact, and another ten to say goodbye, and another ten to tie and untie my boot laces a few times and put my waterproofs on so that no part of me protruded except one eye and one nostril. Finally I stepped outside.

And the rain had stopped. The puddles were full but they were still. The windscreen wipers on the trucks lay flat. I quickly took my waterproofs off before it could start again and we set off for Laddow Rocks, some crags to the north up Crowden Brook.

It had been a fine walk down into this valley the previous evening and it was another one up and out as the path climbed steadily between flanks that rose like something out of Nordic legend. The fresh air was a lubricant and we got into our stride. Boogie seemed to become playful even. I found a tennis ball and I threw it up the path for him and he actually chased after it, something he never normally did. 'One day and you're already rejuvenated!' I chuckled. 'I haven't told you this but they laughed when I said you were going to walk the Pennine Way. They said you weren't up to it, said you were past your prime, said you were. . . .' He had picked up the ball, walked to the cliff edge and dropped it over. We both watched it bounce and fall and lodge in rocks below, and he sat there, all frothy tongue and green teeth, and an expression that said, 'your turn.'

I weighed up the dangers of retrieving the ball against the boost to morale. If I could clamber down there a bond between dog and master would be irreversibly forged. And it wasn't that far down, just a tricky bit in the middle.

Boogie sat and watched, wagged his tail, barked. He seemed eager to sit back and watch me risk my life. I took off my pack and picked my way backwards down the rocks. This was pretty stupid, this was very stupid. I could be the first person to die playing throw and fetch.

I inched down, kicking pebbles and watching them fall hundreds of feet. I reached the ball lodged in a cleft; picked it out and had time to admire the glacial drift that the valley below demonstrated, a fine example of what retreating ice can do given the chance. Rocky crags gave way to slopes as steep as a tub; the valley was green and smooth as a golf course.

I clambered back up, my feet slipping, my nails breaking. I looked up at Boogie, sitting there drooling, looking like he knew something I didn't. Of course the little bastard had staged this to get the insurance.

One big haul and I pulled myself up on to the path. 'There,' I said, and lobbed the ball back to him, and he rolled it straight back down over the cliff again.

* * *

The path climbed gently but inevitably towards the unearthly and unforgiving morass of Black Hill. For such an inhospitable place enough people seemed to have walked up here, enough to cause more erosion problems and for flagstones to have been laid. The work was in progress and a helicopter had dumped dressed slabs of stone in piles along the side of the trail. It was the kind of project that you felt you ought to be lending a hand with. If each walker on the Pennine Way carried one of the flagstones to the end of the line the job would soon be done.

A watery sun came out and shone on the beer-bellied hill, with the path winding up it visible far ahead. The walking was no effort, just a case of picking a way through the wet patches. I walked contemplating mud, and if you're into mud then the Pennine Way is the holiday for you. Having spent the morning crossing a sandstone cocktail, we were now back to our old friend peat, mud of a much more classical texture, and I was beginning to realise that the best way to cope with peat isn't to complain about it, but celebrate it. Peat so often comes in for abuse, but it's succulent, rich, full-bodied stuff with a powerful bouquet, and a good bog is viscous and inky black. You'd pay a fortune for this sort of stuff down a garden centre. I felt tempted to fill a bag with it and post it home for my perennials.

A figure was coming down the slope, moving fast, dancing from rock to rock, and he was quickly upon me. He was walking to Edale in a day, he said, although he looked to me as though he was running. 'My girlfriend's meeting me at the other end,' he puffed excitedly.

I asked him what Black Hill was like and he shook his head and said: 'It's a morass. It's unearthly.'

'Unforgiving?'

'Very unforgiving. You've got to be careful. Keep to the

west of the summit. You'll be in it up to your knees.
You're not supposed to do it alone.'

This was what I had expected to hear, but then he asked
me what Bleaklow was like, and I was about to tell him
it was no trouble at all, and that the path was joined by a
yellow dotted line of paving slabs, and Kinder Scout was
just as straightforward, but before I could help myself I
was saying: 'well, it's tricky. It's an unearthly sort of place.
You've got to concentrate. Trust your compass. Follow
the riverbeds or you'll have trouble.' And as I watched
him jog on down the slope, I told myself that my fiction
was excusable because there was a mythology here that had
to be perpetuated, in case the beast of these moors did wake
up with a headache and turn nasty, and if walkers didn't do
it then no-one would.

As it was, the path up Black Hill was soggy rather
than boggy. The worst moments were when I put my
foot down and felt the whole earth around me sigh and
shudder like something living, and I realised I was on a raft
of vegetation that was slowly sinking under my weight.
And Boogie got a ducking once when he left the path to
chase a bird. One minute he was running over firm peat,
the next he was just a nose sticking out above a swamp.
If Black Hill had had a Hilton, he would have checked
right in.

Otherwise the going was steady and there were always
good views if you walked backwards. And when I turned
to face the front again there was the fabled morass just a
few hundred yards ahead. I'd expected a couple of false
summits, but here was the top of the dome, and I couldn't
believe how dry it looked.

Everyone had said I would never make it to the trig
point here, it wasn't even worth trying. The worst tales
of Black Hill involve walkers who have been airlifted out
of the bog as they've attempted to reach this point, The

Soldiers Lump as it is known. But the surface looked so firm I thought I must have a go.

I put my toe in to test it. I threw a stone for Boogie in the hope he'd run across, and he looked at me as if to say: you think I was born yesterday? I edged towards the middle, as if I was crossing a frozen pond, expecting the ice to crack any moment. But then I was there, clutching onto the concrete stump, The Soldiers Lump, and I felt so pleased with myself I sat down and leaned against it, took my boots off and had my sandwiches.

'Black Hill is a picnic,' I said out loud, and surveyed the view back towards Kinder Scout, now dipping below the horizon. I came over all sentimental and tried to retrace how I had ended up on top of this hill after forty-two years. I felt such a free spirit up here, and yet there was a ball of string in my pocket that linked me helplessly with what I'd left behind. Up here on this bare cap of mud I felt suddenly vulnerable and became conscious of how powerful this terrain was, and how whenever I stopped and looked at it properly I quickly felt a chill and always felt exposed. I was like some fly on a bald head who could be swatted whenever the God of the peat bogs felt bored. What had that walker said earlier: 'you shouldn't be doing this on your own.' So how come he was on his own?

I ate a packet of crisps and you could have heard the crunch in Rochdale. The packet was red, plain. Was red the colour of plain? No. Red was the colour of something much more exciting. Plain crisps should be in a white packet. Red crisps ought to contain something hot. Tabasco flavour. I'd write to them.

The wind was picking up. I looked at Boogie and saw he was sucking on a bone. 'Where the hell did you get that?' I said, and an image came to mind that I was sitting on a pile of dead hikers buried alive in the peat. 'Let's get out of here.'

*   *   *

From this lofty point the land fell sharply away, and the towns of South Yorkshire became visible on the northern horizon. They were the first suggestion that the trial-by-peat we had been subjected to for two days was coming to an end.

There was Holmfirth and there was Huddersfield, and they were spread over country that looked much more hospitable. I stopped and stared when I saw a collection of trees in the distance. They looked like features from a landscape I used to know. The bare moorland of these first two days had been so intense that emerging into this comparative garden I felt a sublime sense of relief, and now with the sun out, shining on the distant glass and metal, these towns looked like resorts.

The moors could change mood with a puff of wind though. One minute they were sunlit and cheery with birdsong. The next the sun would go behind a cloud and an iciness would spike the air and they'd become dark and foreboding again, as now the distant view of civilisation dipped behind a hill and I looked on the map and saw the name Saddleworth Moor. And we all know what happened on Saddleworth Moor.

I emerged on a road and stopped for a cup of tea at a mobile cafe parked in a layby. The owner had a shiny Volvo to pull his caravanette and seemed to be doing very nicely. He threw a ginger nut to Boogie who flicked it up with his nose and caught it in his teeth. Maradona and a football, Boogie and a biscuit, there's no difference.

'Two pullover day, this is,' said the owner as a gust of wind rattled his little café. 'We've had a couple of Pennine Way types through here already. Fit couple of lads, came from Liverpool. They wouldn't have sugar in their tea or anything.'

A van pulled up and a man climbed out and stretched

his arms, showing off the split in his jacket armpit. We both stood and watched the action in the sky. Clouds hurtled across, hurrying as if they were due somewhere else, had to be in London for a dinner appointment at 7.30. They hauled great trains of shadows over the hills. The man said: 'When I win the lottery, the first thing I'm going to do is get myself on one of those cruises, the QE2 or something. Get some decent weather. A friend of my brothers went on the QE2 and he said they used to have midnight buffets and the like.'

I asked him if he'd ever won anything on the lottery and he said: 'not yet. But I used to live in Warrington, where that bloke who won 12 million came from.'

We pressed on to Wissenden Reservoirs and followed the stairway of water down. Reservoirs often found themselves on the front of tourist brochures but they were dour affairs with a Victorian formality that never allowed them to be part of the countryside the way a lake was. They looked temporary, as if you only needed to find a plug to pull and they'd be gone.

What they did do though was underline the fact that despite the wild nature of these moors, we were never far from conurbations of considerable size. In the corner of every view since I'd left home had been a reservoir, or a troop of power pylons striding out from base, or a TV transmission mast. The desolate nature of these moors meant that they had been abandoned and were useful only as a store of resources for the huge populations that lay below them. The sprawl of Greater Manchester was just beyond that hill to the west. Huddersfield, Bradford and Leeds to the east, and these moors were their back yards.

Five o'clock came round again, the time when the soul sinks lowest, when the day seems about to fall off the edge, and on the stroke the sky grew that familiar dirty brown and I felt immediately weary. Boogie stopped at another stile and sat waiting for me to pick him up. I felt like a rant: 'You ought to be getting the message that I'm growing tired of doing this. I have lifted you over 38 stiles since Edale. Look! Stiles are not difficult. Stiles are easy in fact. Stiles are just a case of taking a step up and step down. Watch me. See. I'll do it again for you. A step up and a step. . . .'

I fell silent as a walker approached. I hadn't seen him scrambling down rocks off the path, and now he was very close and smiling at me, smiling at the nutter demonstrating stiles to his dim dog. He was dressed entirely in blue, but as he reached me I could see his bottom half was stained dark brown. He'd been up to his waist in something.

'Just fallen in a bog,' he said proudly, as if his day had been worthwhile now. I looked down at myself. I was very clean and tidy still. My boots had dried and I had no muck around my chin like he did. I felt like a virgin. He looked at me and no doubt pictured my car parked at the top of the hill.

'Your dog's nice and dirty anyway,' he said and walked off.

Boogie was dirty indeed. Dirty and smelly with bog-water. I was going to look for lodgings soon and no landlady would have fancied the idea of Boogie lying on her hearth rug. As we passed a peaceful moorland waterfall I turned it into a violent one by shoving Boogie underneath and giving him a shower. 'Help! Pet being abused!' he barked as he went under for the third time.

I found another bunkhouse that night, in another little community very similar to Crowden the previous evening, neatly lined up along a trans-Pennine trunk road with juggernauts steaming past the window in the mist. The woman opened the door to me and said, 'It's dog night tonight isn't it?'

She meant there were two other men staying with dogs, and that wasn't all. 'There's also a party of people with learning difficulties,' she whispered. 'I thought I'd better tell you.'

My bed had a Union Jack pillow, and all over the walls were notices in fluorescent pen: 'People caught washing with the tap running will be shot.' 'Someone has to clean up, why not you?'

I fed Boogie and he lay down and looked at me with what I took to be a happy smile but in fact was the face of a dog asleep with his eyes open. I prodded him awake. 'This isn't the dog I used to know,' I said. 'What happened to the socialite who never came in until the last curry house had closed. Let's go and paint the village red.'

We walked up the road to find the pub. The fog was so bad I wondered if I should have brought my compass. I shivered when I thought of what it must be like now back up on Black Hill.

Trucks loomed out of the vapour and moaned their way down the hill, all lights and screaming gears. The village was a group of houses where innocent people sat waiting for a runaway juggernaut to bulldoze into their living room in the middle of Panorama.

I bumped into a big building and I ran my hands along until I found the pub front door. Inside, the landlord was standing behind his pumps, beaming. He said, 'Been walking the Pennine Way?'

'Yes.'

'I could tell.'

'How could you tell?'

'I can just tell. Those two over there have been walking the Pennine Way. You can tell that as well.'

I looked and there were two men with moustaches sitting at a table with their arms folded, and under their feet two knackered dogs. One was a huge rottweiler, the other was a labrador.

'Another bloke on the Pennine Way,' the landlord called out to them. They made room for me and I sat down and folded my arms in solidarity. Boogie sat underneath with the rottweiler and labrador and tuned into their dreams.

'Staying at the Bunk house?' the man with the labrador asked.

'Yes,' I said

'So are we,' said the lad with the rottweiler

We sat and supped our pints. 'Black Hill was terrible wasn't it?' asked rottweiler-man.

'Unearthly,' I said.

'A morass,' said labrador-man.

I complained of the weight of dog food in my pack: 'I'm carrying a three kilo bag.'

'I'm carrying a five kilo,' said the labrador.

'I'm carrying a pack for my stuff on my back and a pack for dog food on my front,' said the rottweiler.

I told them about Boogie and stiles, how I had to lift him over. 'He weighs three stone,' I said.

The rottweiler and labrador had the same problem. 'My dog weighs four and a half,' said the labrador.

'Seven,' said the rottweiler. 'But he's losing weight.'

They say people resemble their dogs but these two looked like each other's dog. The man with the rottweiler had big ears and a square head and shiny black hair. The man with the labrador had dark eyes, big teeth and no neck.

'So what are you walking the Pennine Way for?' asked the rottweiler.

'I thought the dog needed a good walk,' I said

'Same here,' said the rottweiler.

'Same here,' said the labrador. 'It's the kind of walk he's always wanted to do.'

'. . . and so I thought I'd do it with him while he still could,' said the rottweiler.

'Me too,' I said.

'He needed a challenge,' said the labrador.

'Exactly,' said the rottweiler.

'A challenge, exactly,' I said.

'Is yours enjoying it?' asked the labrador.

'Oh he's loving it,' I said

'So's mine,' said the rottweiler.

'He was just sitting at home doing nothing.'

'So was mine.'

'Mine too.'

We supped our pints. One of the dogs farted. 'I think that was mine,' said the labrador.

'No it was mine,' I said.

'It wasn't mine,' said the rottweiler. 'You'd know if it was mine.'

The labrador leant forward and said quietly, 'You know what I've heard? There are Pennine Way groupies.'

'Getaway,' said the rottweiler.

'That's what I've been told,' said the labrador. 'There are women who hang about round the camp sites and hostels on the path and pick up blokes who are walking the Pennine Way.'

There was a silence as we all imagined what it would be like to be propositioned by a Pennine Way groupie. None of us much liked the idea.

'Who told you that?' I asked.

'Friend of my brother's who's walked it,' said the labrador. 'Said it happened to him.'

'Where?' asked the rottweiler.

'Near Hadrian's Wall.'

I said, 'You don't associate the Pennine Way with sex, do you?'

'You don't,' said the rottweiler.

'You associate it with mud and damp,' I said.

'And misery,' said the labrador.

'And dog biscuit,' said the rottweiler.

We supped our pints.

'I bet you can count on one hand the number of people who have scored on the Pennine Way,' said the rottweiler.

We all looked so tired sitting there. Red rims round our eyes, ruddy faces, trying to keep back the yawns. The labrador said, 'we were just talking about negative equity before you came along. How it screws everything up, all your plans. I blame the failure of my marriage on negative equity. . . .'

Back at the bunkhouse the group with learning difficulties had arrived. They'd been out all day at a market and now they wandered round in shirts and no trousers. One lad was standing up against the wall saying, 'You mustn't play with water. You're a naughty boy to play with water.' He saw me and said, 'My name is Roger, what's yours?'

'Mark.'

'I like dogs. Dogs like me.' And he patted Boogie into the ground.

He took me into the common room to meet his friends. I tried to make conversation, but I couldn't think what to say to them. I found myself speaking slowly and loudly, and soon I felt exhausted. I went to phone home. Catherine took a while to answer. She said, 'I fell asleep putting the children to bed.'

Roger passed in the corridor. 'You mustn't play with water. You're a naughty boy to play with water.'

I talked to Catherine about peat for a while. I was surprised at how much I had to say on the subject. I asked how the kids were and she said, 'Francis thinks

you've been eaten by a dinosaur and Daniel thinks you've
gone to the pub.'

Roger and his friends made a lot of noise and kept me
awake until past midnight. I read *Wuthering Heights* and
fell into a fitful sleep, dreaming helplessly. I dreamed I
was walking over springy peat bogs and other walkers
were waving and calling to me, and when I looked down
at myself I was naked apart from my boots.

I woke because a voice was outside my door. Heathcliffe,
I thought, as *Wuthering Heights* slipped over the bed and
onto Boogie's head. But it was Roger. He was talking
in his monotone: 'I must not go into rooms unless I am
invited. I must not play with water and I must not go into
rooms unless I am invited.'

I saw the man with the rottweiler leave the next morning
very early, the mist creeping over the moors like a drug.
. He did have two packs, a huge one on his back and
one on his front that was smaller, but probably only so he
could see over the top. The big dog marched in front on
a chain. They looked like hiker and pack animal suffering
from role reversal.

I came down for breakfast and there were the two men
from Liverpool. 'Are you sure you're not walking the
Pennine Way?' asked Doug.

'Sure,' I said.

They had a room in the main house. 'It's *en suite*,'
said Tony.

'It's very clean,' said Doug

'Where's your dog?' asked Tony

'Upstairs studying a bus timetable.'

Their stories unfolded between mouthfuls of full English
breakfast. They were workmates. Doug was my age; Tony
was in his fifties. Tony had always wanted to walk the
Pennine Way. He'd promised himself he'd do it when

he retired, but his wife had urged him to go while he was still fit.

Tony said, 'He's got a problem with his prostate.'

Doug blushed: 'Do you mind?'

'Nothing to be ashamed of.'

'I don't go telling people about your vasectomy, do I?'

'You can tell who you like about my vasectomy,' said Tony.

'We were just talking about backpacks actually,' said Doug, trying to change the subject. 'The different weight distribution that a Berghaus offers compared to a Karrimor.'

But Tony was happy to talk to me about his vasectomy. 'It's just a nip and a tuck you know, the operation, nothing to worry about. The increased risk of testicular cancer is too insignificant to be a factor. You can't ride a horse for a while afterwards, that's all.'

The woman brought in more toast. We all refused but she said, 'You want to eat lots of toast if you're walking the Pennine Way,' and so we all took a slice.

She stood in the doorway and complained about the pub up the road: 'Seventeen years we've lived here and now that new bloke arrives and wants to open all day.'

'Opening all day doesn't work,' her husband said, joining her in the kitchen doorway. 'What it means is the walkers stay too long up there and have too much to drink and then come back here for their supper and complain the food's overcooked. You can't keep roast potatoes hot, you know.'

He cleared the table and disappeared into the kitchen and came back again and never once stopped talking. He was trying to be chatty but he ended up moaning. 'I fell out with one Pennine Way couple over roast potatoes. I said to them: "get your bloody arse down the road to the hotel. This is my house. You're just guests."'

He realised he had raised his voice and now he looked

embarrassed. 'More toast,' he said. 'You need to eat toast if you're walking the Pennine Way.' And so we all took more toast.

The bunkhouse had been warm and damp, and climbing up onto the moors again, I came the nearest I'm ever likely to come to experiencing what washing feels when it's put out on a blustery day. You couldn't imagine the wind ever dropping up here. The gusts got in my pockets and I sailed up to Millstone Edge. Ammon Wrigley, the poet and writer of local folklore, loved this place so much a plaque commemorating his life has been placed here and his ashes scattered, although it's unlikely any of them hit the ground before the wind got hold of them and blew them back into Rochdale.

It was a morning of walking on top of the world, and when the mist cleared the excellent visibility of the previous two days returned and the views tumbled far away to where urban areas sat coughing in clouds of bus fumes. The pylons and reservoirs still made you feel connected to these cities but you felt safe up here. You filled your lungs with freshly laundered air and felt lucky. Boogie stood on a crag with his ears blown out at right angles and looked longingly down to the flesh pots of Oldham.

The path stuck to the rim of the moor, the peat creeping to the edge like a lava flow. I walked on wondering if I'd ever have a plaque dedicated to me. It was unlikely. I needed to invent something, something unique, something that bore my name: a raincoat like Mr Mackintosh; a traffic beacon like Mr Belisha; something that turned me into an overnight eponym, so people would say, 'can I borrow your Wallington, mine's broken.' Or, 'guess what I bought Grandma for Christmas? A new Wallington.' Or even, 'cor! those Wallington's are tasty today.'

A Wallington could be a device that you point at shirts

and it irons them automatically? Or a shoe that fits either foot so you can buy them singly and not worry if you lose one?

Time flies when you're enjoying yourself. Before I knew it, we were striding into Yorkshire, towards the M62 and another snack caravan waiting by the sliproad. This was Brian's, and I would suggest he serves the best fruit pasties in the Pennines. I told him I was walking the Pennine Way and he asked, 'Are you enjoying it?'

'Yes, thank you.'

'Your dog isn't, is he?'

'Yes he is.'

'How come he looks so fed up?'

'He's not fed up. He's got that sort of face.'

'What sort of face?'

'An ironic face.'

Boogie was looking with great irony at the M62, wondering if he could climb up on that bridge and jump down on a passing truck and stow away to somewhere where they understood bone-idle dogs.

Brian said he got walkers from all nations stopping at his snack bar. 'German, American, Canadian, and that other place. Used to be lots more than there are now.'

A round man climbed out of his car and hoisted his trousers up. Brian said to him: 'Back from Lancaster already?'

Crossing these major roads, it always felt odd to look at the cars and trucks and think that they could be in Scotland by the afternoon if they put their foot down, in the kind of time it would take me to walk to the next village. Someone like this tubby man with loose trousers had been to Lancaster, done a morning's work and come back again, and it was only lunchtime. He had a fruit pastie and a tea and leant on the counter. 'I'm off to bloody where-do-you-call-it next.'

'Where?' asked Brian.

'That place with concrete cows.'

'Milton Keynes,' I said.

'Aye.' And he climbed in his car and sat there looking at the traffic.

'What does he do?' I asked Brian.

'I've never found out,' said Brian. 'The Dutch, those are the fellas. They like the Pennine Way as well. 'Cos it's flat where they live you see. I can always tell the Dutch as they come over that hill.'

Brian pointed me towards the footbridge across the M62, the bridge that had to be built for walkers because the motorway crossed a right of way. It reminded me of the tunnels that constructors dug when their new roads crossed an ancient badger thoroughfare. It was as if Pennine Way walkers were powered by instinct, and without this bridge they'd have had no choice but to climb the fence and walk blindly across the motorway, and end up as roadkill.

As it is the bridge is a fine vantage point and if you're feeling withdrawal symptoms after three relatively traffic-free days you can stand here and look down into the cockpits of cars and lorries and inhale motorway culture at its best. Drivers in suits, drivers in vests, drivers in short skirts, drivers in long skirts. Drivers slapping their knees to music, slapping their passenger's knee to music. Drivers picking their nose, picking their passenger's nose.

The volume is huge and the impact the motorway makes enormous. It is worth remembering though that the M62 is just the latest in a succession of roads that has crossed these hills for as long as there have been communities on either side, so that military ways, packhorse trails, turnpikes and now motorways often run parallel to, or in some cases on top of, one another. Not far from here, running up to Blackstone Edge, is a good example of this, where an old trans-Pennine route, disused for many years, can be seen well-preserved.

I'd read it was up here somewhere just off the path and I spent a while hunting round. Then when I found it — an impressive black, rutted causeway — I couldn't think of anything to do but sit and have lunch on its gritstone cobbles. I closed my eyes and tried to recreate the scene, the kind that TV brings to life with such ease as mists clear and the sound of hooves and carriages fades in, and suddenly people in costume are trotting past, lifting their top hats.

I jumped as something landed in my lap, a tennis ball, and I looked up to see Boogie standing over me, strangely playful again, with a 'go on, throw it for me and I'll do a backward somersault like those stunt dogs on Blue Peter do' look on his face. I pretended to throw the ball for him and he got confused and sniffed round for it, spent ages sniffing round for it in fact. Poor sad dog.

I leaned back against a rock in the sun and listened to the radio. Wednesday afternoon and I was sitting by an ancient road wandering through the airwaves, the feeling of guilt at having nothing to do but walk growing weaker. The news came on, details of the various murders committed in the north west. Two men from Liverpool were wanted for questioning. The bulletin was hardly over when I heard voices coming down the path, and peered out of my cranny to see my two friends from Liverpool striding north.

'He bought himself a fleece and a pair of waterproof trousers for £25. . . .' said Doug

'Never,' said Tony.

'It's true!' said Doug.

'You're making that up.'

'I'm not making it up.'

I couldn't imagine these two as murderers somehow. Murder victims maybe.

They didn't see me and I waited a while to let them get ahead. But then as soon as I came out from behind my rock there was another walker coming down the path, a man

travelling north to south. You could tell this simply because
he had a brown face and a peeling nose whereas the vast
majority of walkers on the Pennine Way, those travelling
south to north, had sunburnt necks. He didn't slow as he
approached and he would probably have walked straight
past me with just a nod if I hadn't blocked the path.

He mumbled a greeting.

'Walking the Pennine Way?' I said.

He sighed and said yes, he was.

'A north to souther. Don't meet many of them.'

'No.'

I asked him if he'd seen the two men from Liverpool and
he said he had and they'd asked him where he'd bought his
compass and what price he paid for it.

He wanted to get moving. He said: 'the trouble with
walking north to south is that you have to stop and talk
to all the people going south to north and they ask you
such stupid questions.'

'Oh,' I said, and tried to think of a sensible question.
'Why are you doing it north to south?'

'That's what everyone asks me.'

He was doing it north to south because he'd done it
south to north years ago and he knew that Kirk Yetholm,
the village at the end of the Pennine Way, was a dead
end. 'The hardest part of the Pennine Way, if you want
my opinion, is getting out of Kirk Yetholm. The place is
a dump.'

And with that he strode off.

'So,' I said to Boogie, 'we're walking 276 miles just to
end up in a dump.'

The path headed for Hebden Bridge, winding round more
reservoirs on a firm gravel track that allowed us to get into a
steady rhythm and eat up the miles. The peat bogs seemed
far behind me now. On Bleaklow and Black Hill I'd felt I

had to concentrate, to watch all angles, now I daydreamed, now I slowed and found myself blushing as a chain of thought left me stranded at a point ten years ago, standing on a stage in Austria somewhere, having just volunteered to yodel along with the Hippacher Trio in front of a coach load of tourists from Intasun. Up here on the moors above Calderdale I stared at the ground in embarrassment all over again.

The terrain began to look lived in. A windmill farm waved at me in the distance and I was walking towards a monument on a hill, a huge finger of blackened gritstone known as Stoodley Pike that pointed disapprovingly at the sky.

The wind buffeted it as I struggled to read the eroded inscription on the commemoration plaque. The tower was begun in 1814 to celebrate the end of the Napoleonic Wars, but then Napoleon escaped from Elba a year into construction and so they downed tools. Wellington gave them something else to celebrate with the battle of Waterloo so they started work again and completed the project. It collapsed in 1854.

There was a balcony halfway up and I thought I would get a good view down into Hebden Bridge and Calderdale. A door led to a dark staircase which disappeared into the belly of the monument. I peered inside and took five steps into the blackness. The air was suddenly damp, my boots echoed on the old stone and I could see nothing. Something hairy swung across my face and I turned and hurried outside, and bumped right into a couple of grey-haired ladies wearing breeches and hats with ear mufflers.

'What's the view from the top like?' they asked. They sounded like the sort you'd meet on the North Downs out for the air.

'Oh it's wonderful,' I said.

'You've got a spider in your hair,' said one.

'Yes I know. Thanks.'

They disappeared into the passage. I heard them climb the stairs and then saw them reappear high on the balcony with their hands shading their eyes looking down into the valley.

'You and your dog look as though you're walking the Pennine Way,' one woman called down to me.

'We are,' I replied and tried to look enigmatic as I turned and headed down into Hebden Bridge.

'Did you hear that, Boogie? We look as though we're walking the Pennine Way. That's good. That's marvellous. I think.'

And he looked up at me to say, 'All right. I give up. I can't find that tennis ball.'

3. Quiz Night in Brontë Country

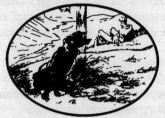

The steep path from the moors into Hebden Bridge was like going down in a department store elevator.

Top floor: windswept moorland, sheep, curlew, big sky.

Third floor: farmland, cattle, barns, rattle of tractors.

Second floor: woodland, streams, song birds.

First floor: residential, washing strung across street.

Ground floor: canalside, cafés, museum of myths, legends and horrors.

The woodland was dappled with sunlight, the moss green as a snooker table and so sweet-smelling after three days having my senses blasted on the moors. I whistled my way down the line of trees into the valley until we emerged on the Rochdale canal and followed the towpath towards town.

Here were backyards and kids playing in sandboxes; bean-poles in back gardens, the sizzle of the evening meal. It was so much warmer at this level, and every kitchen window was flung open in welcome. It felt like a homecoming from some foreign country. The string of geese blocking the path ahead waddled up and down like customs officials.

There was no way round them and when they saw Boogie they stiffened and prepared for trouble. I was at a loss how to tackle them but then I saw a sign in a window that said, 'Clap your hands and the geese will go away.' So I self-consciously clapped my hands, and in response the geese gave me long necks and hisses, quite the opposite of going away.

I clapped my hands again, more loudly, and I may have growled. They didn't go away again. So I said: 'Shoo!' And they blew raspberries at me.

I hoped no-one was watching me being humiliated by a few motley geese. I'd have offered them money if I'd thought they would have taken it. I needed to be assertive. I needed to charge them, show them who was in control. Better still Boogie could charge them. 'Do something,' I said.

Do something yourself, he grunted.

Then just as I was about to get tough, they waddled away down the side of the house as if it was time for Neighbours.

I had a friend in Hebden Bridge who had offered to put me up, and so soon I was sitting at a kitchen table, drinking mugs of tea, my backpack leaning against the couch I was to sleep on.

Boogie couldn't find the television so he stared at the washing machine all evening, leaving me to recount the journey so far to Sarah. I told her how Bleaklow was hell on earth, how I didn't think I'd get off Black Hill alive, and she said, 'So how come you look so clean and tidy?'

I didn't know why I looked so clean and tidy. I looked as though I'd just spent the day in the office rather than on the Pennine Way. I resembled one of those models in the outdoor clothing magazines. I said, 'Maybe I'm doing something wrong. I haven't even got wet yet. Three days on the Pennine Way and no rain.'

As I spoke hail hit the windows like gravel. 'Look what you've gone and done now,' said Sarah, and she ran outside to pull the laundry off the line. I went to help her and the whole street was out in backyards and gardens grabbing at laundry.

'The weather is very temperamental in Hebden Bridge,' she said, back inside. 'You don't want to annoy it by saying things like: three days on the Pennine Way and no rain.'

She took me on a walking tour of the town the next morning, and anyone who lives in Hebden Bridge could probably walk the Pennine Way with a bag of shopping on each arm, so steep are the streets. It's hard to walk anywhere without going up.

But this means it's a town of many fine views. Climb any of the hillsides and you can look down into the cramped valley and imagine what it looked like in its industrial heyday, and realise what a damn sight better looking place it is now.

That heyday was at the turn of the century, during the cotton mill boom, when everyone in Calderdale was involved in textiles in one way or another. No-one knows how many mills there were in Hebden Bridge at that time, but old pictures show a jungle of chimneys and a smog so dense it makes you feel churlish to complain about poor air quality today. They say the smoke used to get worse as the week got on. 'I could tell what day of the week it was by the thickness of the smog' is one reminiscence.

In such a narrow valley, space in the bottom was at a premium and every square foot was taken up by mills and industrial premises. When the town needed dwelling space it could only build up the steep slopes, so that now it looks as though it's stacked on shelving.

The further up you go the grander are the houses. Back-to-backs on the bottom and villas on the top. And in between, the strange under-and-over dwellings: houses with six storeys, the bottom three fronting on one street and comprising one home, and the top three fronting on the next street up, and comprising home number two.

The boom years in Hebden Bridge saw a turnpike road built, then a canal – the first waterway through the Pennines – and then the railway steamed through as Calderdale became a channel for industry and communications.

It flourished until after the First World War, but by then foreign imports had begun to compete with homespun business and inevitably recession set in. The town fell into decline, only held together by its own grime. Not until the Seventies did it show any sign of recovery, when hippies moved in and it gained a bohemian cachet. Then the hippies grew up and became yuppies. Estate agents and tourism took over and the town began to prosper again. Now it's riding on the wave of industrial heritage. Most of the old mills have been converted into homes or arcades or industrial units. Art galleries, cafés, and museums have emerged out of the dinosaur-like ruins of the old days. A liberal spirit flourishes. A man chalked up the menu on a pub blackboard, and turned to me and asked 'How the hell do you spell asparagus?'

The town had a glow to it on that bright morning. The hillsides dripped with sunlight and the washing was out again, hanging across the streets like bunting. On Windsor Road and Broughton Street a few signs of the hippy era existed still. The laundry was tie-dyed and the drainpipes were painted in rainbow colours. A few greying pony tails bounced down the street.

It seemed like a dreamy place to live, and yet under the surface a nightmare had come to life. The town was still holding its head as it recovered from the murder of a young local girl. She'd gone missing one evening the previous November, and not been found until the spring when workers dredging the canal pulled out her stone-weighted body. She'd been strangled.

This seemed such a tight community that even reading about this terrible affair in the local newspaper made me feel like an intruder. People got used to hearing about murders on the radio, committed in some distant place they'd never been to, but when one happened on their own doorstep it didn't slip away with yesterday's news. It ingrained itself in the town, lurked behind every façade, sat at the back of everyone's mind. What made matters worse was that police were apparently convinced a local man, someone who knew the victim, was responsible.

I climbed the hill up to Heptonstall, the original village from which the bigger industrial community grew, and from here there were wonderful views over the town. You could see how everything leaned towards the eponymous bridge at its centre. A woman with three young children sat down on the bench and said, 'Who wants their nose blown?'

This pleasant town with nice shops and nice people and, somewhere among them, quite possibly a murderer.

Sarah suggested she walk with me out of town through a wooded ravine named Hardcastle Crags. This meant missing out a section of Pennine Way, but the crags were a local attraction and I liked the idea of staying in the shelter of this valley for as long as I could.

Boogie wanted to stay in the shelter of Sarah's house for as long as he could. I'd let him lie in all morning while I walked round town, and when I returned and hoisted my pack on my back again, he looked at me as though I was crazy, like: we've got a good deal going in this house. There's a comfy couch and there are domestic appliances. There's a cat to chase down the street. What do you want to go and spoil things for?

Now he walked behind Sarah and me, wishing he'd raided the fridge while we were out.

Hardcastle Crags was a tunnel of woodland, so dense in foliage it hid the crags for which it was known. In times past this was a very popular beauty spot. Charabancs of trippers from the factories would come on outings to Gibson Mill, where there were facilities for dancing and roller skating. Now the mill was boarded up and had weeds growing out of the stone. It looked odd because from just one morning in Hebden Bridge, it had become evident how closely guarded anything which added to the wealth of the local heritage was. You got the feeling there would be a museum of something or other in this redundant building before too long.

Sarah left me at Gibson Mill and turned back to town. She said, 'I've always wanted to walk the Pennine Way but didn't think I could manage it. Looking at you, though, I think perhaps I could.'

I headed north, climbing through the glade, back towards the hills. I'd gone a hundred yards before I realised that Boogie had followed Sarah.

'He's a joker, isn't he?' she said. 'A real bundle of laughs.'

I grabbed him and pushed him off up towards open country. He shook his head with a 'You don't understand, do you? This is madness.'

I did understand. Leaving Hebden Bridge was like starting again; a lesson in how deadly it is to get comfortable somewhere, to find a regular place to sit, to know where the teabags are kept, to read a local paper. I had that old knot back in the stomach as I followed signposts up to the moor.

At least I was no longer a freshman, pale and with soft feet. I had a sunburnt neck, damn it, the blues of my eyes were sharpening. I had the face of someone left out in the weather, and I could look back and see the summit of Black Hill with its TV mast just visible to the south, and know that I had come over that.

The sky was as busy as ever. A great wagon train of cloud rumbled overhead, rolling rolling rolling, like some migration east. It started to drizzle and we sheltered in grouse butt no 3 on the Saville Estate. Boogie took this opportunity to eat grass and throw up. My apologies to Lord Saville if this puts him off his shot on the Twelfth of August.

A downpour looked imminent and I pulled my waterproofs out, but as soon as I got an arm into a sleeve, the rain stopped and the cloud blew over and the sun came out. Pretty good waterproofs, I thought. You just shake them at rain clouds and that frightens them off. Even Gore-tex can't do that.

A field of wind turbines had appeared on a slope across the valley. The small cluster I'd seen the previous afternoon had been only the corner of a much larger crop of these strange machines. A lucrative crop too, some local farmers were offering as many acres as they could to Renewable Energy Systems, who would then build wind farms of twenty to thirty turbines.

Local pressure groups had quickly realised the threat to the natural beauty of the countryside. 'Save our Moors from Wind Turbines' the stickers in windows in Hebden Bridge had said. Farmers challenged the environmentalist groups to 'put up or shut up'. They argued they should be left to make the best return on the land that they could.

Hebden Bridge's famous son, Bernard Ingham, writing in the local press, had words to say about that: 'The price of preserving our Pennine Heritage is eternal vigilance and resolute campaigning against resourceful developers and farmers who stand to make a killing . . . If a community

wishes to retain its familiar horizons it will have to fight
for them.'

As I stood on a rise over Walshaw reservoirs and gazed
at the turbines lined up on the hillsides, a fight was what
they appeared to be preparing for. They had the poise of
some military force, stood to attention, tall and resolute.
They looked like the landing of some alien invasion.

I reached the Pennine Way again and it felt like I was
back on the road. This was the highway and paths like
the one from Hebden Bridge were slip roads that travellers
took to and from the suburbs each evening and morning.

Boogie trotted off in the slow lane, but then he was
coming back to me with a prize which he laid at my
feet: a ladies' pink slip. I examined it: St Michael, size
16. 'Where did you get this?' I asked.

He barked, but this was because a walker was coming
down the path, a walker who was already eyeing sus-
piciously the man in front of him holding up a ladies'
undergarment. I couldn't just toss it back in the heather;
nor could I stuff it in my pocket. I suppose I could have
blown my nose on it.

'Mrng,' I said. 'Lovely day for it.

He said nothing: perverts were best ignored.

I pressed on, now with a pink slip in the compartment of
my rucksack normally reserved for lunch. We were back on
moorland, although this was much tamer stuff, well trod,
and civilised by duckboards and literature. There should
have been a sign here really, YOU ARE NOW ENTERING
BRONTË COUNTRY.

I crested a ridge and there ahead was a haunting view of
a ruined farmhouse. No ordinary ruin this, though, this was
Top Withens, a shrine for anyone on the Brontë trail, the
farmhouse that was supposed to have been the inspiration
for the Earnshaw house in *Wuthering Heights*.

I could see two walkers sitting on a wall nearby as I

approached. They were drinking from their flasks and they waved and lifted their cups when they saw me – the Liverpool duo.

We greeted each other with a hiker's nod and shuffle. 'You *are* walking the Pennine Way, aren't you?' said Doug.

'Me? No,' I replied, and sat on the wall with them. 'So this is Top Withens is it?'

'Top Withens it is,' said Doug.

'That's what the book says,' said Tony

I wondered if we should have a literary discussion. I tried to think of something profound to say about *Wuthering Heights* even though I was only up to Page 8. Doug too, sensing that this was a special place, had the decency to look meditative, as though the spirit of Emily Brontë was having a not insignificant effect on him.

Tony looked uncomfortable with this. We sat there in silence for a moment. I peeled an orange. Tony bit his lip, and could resist it no longer. He said to me, 'What sort of boots are those?'

And you could sense the relief all round.

'Brasher boots,' I said.

'I've got Brasher boots,' said Tony.

'So have I,' said Doug. 'They're very good, aren't they?'

'I'm very happy with them,' I said.

I imagined these two meeting the ghost of Emily Brontë striding up to Top Withens and stopping her to ask where she got her jacket. I said, 'Did you know Charlotte Brontë died while still in her thirties, after catching a chill from walking on the moors in the rain?'

'You read that in the guide book, didn't you?' said Doug with a grin.

'Yes,' I said.

'People in those days didn't have the right equipment,' said Tony.

'No,' I said.

'You can get them resoled, and get new eyes and new rims for about twenty-five pounds you know?'

'What?'

'For those Brasher boots. They're very good value.'

They packed up their things and slung their packs on their backs. 'Well, we'll leave you in peace to have your orange,' said Tony.

Top Withens was just a shell and you had to switch your imagination up to 'extra vivid' to conjure up the Brontë connection. And even if you managed to achieve that, one look at the plaque on the wall brought you back to reality with a crunch:

> The buildings, even when complete, bore no resemblance to the house she described [in *Wuthering Heights*] but the situation may have been in her mind when she wrote of the moorland setting.

There was an honesty here that was refreshing and I liked the way the temptation to rebuild the house around Emily Brontë's writing desk or something had been resisted. This was pilgrims' country after all, and they could have got away with an audio-visual display at the very least. Top Withens may have been four miles out of the Brontë centre of Haworth and over rough moorland, but it was on the circumnavigation known as the Brontë Way, and many visitors made it up here. A signpost nearby marked the junction of the Brontë Way and the Pennine Way in five languages, including Japanese. I was so amused, I took a photo.

You could only admire the dedication of these tourists. As I left the Pennine Way once again and followed the

Brontë Way down into Haworth I was passed by all nationalities, battling against the chill wind and ominous sky, holding umbrellas and dressed in the kind of gear that would have had my friends from Liverpool perform citizen's arrests. But they had their heads down and they were going to make it to Brontë Falls and to the Brontë chair and to Top Withens no matter what. They had the driven look of tourists who have already paid for their excursions.

'Is this the way to *Wuthering Heights*?' asked one American, dressed in a short-sleeved shirt and golf shoes – maybe their plan was to die on the moors like Charlotte Brontë.

'That's right,' I said. '*Wuthering Heights*, straight on.'

And then later I got trapped in a kissing gate and two Germans had to rescue me. 'That's a funny looking dog,' said one, which was uncalled for, and a cheek because he was no picture himself.

'He looks like the Hound of the Baskervilles,' said his friend, making me wonder if they really knew which literary trail they were on.

I followed the Brontë Way down into Haworth, annoying myself by singing Kate Bush's *Wuthering Heights* all the way. But it was good to approach such a well-visited place on a footpath rather than a road, and to enter the village through the churchyard. Most people came in via the coach park and never saw the few innocent corners that remained. Once you emerged on the cobbled high street you never got off it. That was Haworth there, rolled out down the hill in all its glory.

It was pleasantly uncrowded when I arrived, just as the shops were closing up. I had the street to myself for a while. You could imagine what a honeypot this was, though. From the Brontë parsonage at the top – which was now a museum owned by the Brontë Society – to the steam train at the bottom, there was hardly a building that hadn't cashed in.

To be blessed with a literary family of the stature of the Brontës as local residents is the kind of endorsement a village dreams about these days. It's even better than being chosen as a location for a TV series. Classical novelists have longevity; they breed economic confidence and long-term investment, and attract a better class of tourist. This may sound cynical but it's hard to be anything else in a village where they wear period costume in the chemists.

I saw only one Japanese though, a man reading the Yorkshire pudding recipe on a tea towel in a gift shop. Maybe the rest were all indoors watching their compatriot on TV playing tennis in the French Open. The woman who ran the B&B where I stopped, switched it on when I arrived. She said, 'We used to get a lot of Japanese here, but they've got unemployment in their country now.' She showed me her visitors' book. 'See, we get visitors from all over. We had a gentleman from Belgium the other night.' She emphasised the word gentleman as though everyone else who came from Belgium was a hooligan.

Later Boogie and I strolled back up the hill through the public gardens heading for the quiz night at The Bull. Making sure no-one was looking I nonchalantly deposited a ladies' pink slip in a bin.

On the road a bus pulled up. The doors hissed open and Boogie tugged to jump on board. He does this instinctively to every bus but then when I saw the word Bradford on the front I thought: you know what would really make this evening memorable? The whiff of a curry floated into my head and I couldn't resist it.

'How long does it take to Bradford?' I asked the driver. 'Forty minutes.'

Forty-five minutes later I was waiting in the Kashmir Restaurant in Bradford for a takeaway. The only diner in hiking boots. I took my order outside where the strangely well-behaved and ever faithful Boogie was waiting with the biggest smile I'd seen on his face since Edale. We sat on a bench and split a portion of Pakal dahl and chapattis.

Above us, on a billboard, the dog from the complete dog food advert looked back: square jaw, muscular neck, a Hollywood smile. 'Don't worry. You're getting there,' I said to Boogie. 'He smells of Old Spice, you smell of silage, that's the only difference.'

We finished the curry and I went back in and asked for the same again. The waiter said, 'Hungry boy.'

'I'm walking the Pennine Way,' I told him.

'Really?'

'Yes.'

'Of course you are,' he beamed. The customer is always right even if he's nutty enough to claim he's walking the Pennine Way.

I sat there cocooned in this dark and spicy place with calendars on every wall, thinking: if you're walking the Pennine Way and you find yourself in a curry house in Bradford, then surely things are going seriously wrong. I began to panic. Outside I hurried through my meal, and after a quick visit to an Asian sweet shop, we jumped back on a bus to Haworth.

Which was all a shame, because later as I sat in The Bull among the strange collection of contestants at the quiz night – walkers, Brontë pilgrims, businessmen from Holland, all trying to think who was the original host of *The Generation Game* – it struck me that, above all, the Pennine Way is a journey through the north of England, and the image I'd had that day of it being a highway and all other paths leading off and onto it had been a good one. You can put your head down and walk its length and impress yourself with a show of stamina, but it's much more interesting to use the path as a thread, and to come off it at

any point that takes your fancy and have a taste of whatever
is available. If the Pennine Way was good enough to offer
me a good curry then it would have been ungrateful of me
to turn it down.

Then when I got back to my lodgings I switched on
the TV and the news was just breaking of riots in Bradford
that night – race riots. A police patrol had tried to break
up a gang of Asian youths and in the process manhandled
a protesting Asian woman and driven their car over
someone's foot. The tension between the police and Asian
community, strained at the best of times, had snapped.

Spending all day walking, it was easy to stick your head
in the clouds and imagine the Pennines were nothing but
moors and dales and small communities. But they were also
big cities and people who had never seen a peat bog. If the
Pennine Way is a journey through the north of England
then maybe a visit to Bradford should be on every walker's
itinerary.

A man in overalls climbed out from under his Austin,
and pointed his spanner down the lane. 'You want to
turn left just past the bridge and follow the old packhorse
trail. . . .'

I got a thrill every time someone said, 'follow that
packhorse trail'. I saw fifty horses piled with lead or
salt or fish, their bells ringing as they travelled up and
over the moor in all weathers. For five hundred years,
until the turnpike roads were introduced, packhorses were
the only means of transporting freight in these parts, and
walking on the Pennine Way, evidence of the routes
they followed is never far away. Everyday you come
across one of the unmistakable narrow bridges, just wide
enough for a horse to cross; or you pass a Packhorse
Inn like the one near Widdop; or, as on this morning,
the Pennine Way actually followed one of the trails.

'Mush,' I said to Boogie, and he turned and stuck his tongue out at me.

Ahead a shepherd and his dog were at work, wheeling their sheep, a perfect team. That was the kind of spirit I'd have liked to generate between Boogie and me, but he's not that kind of animal. The years have turned him into a cynic. I knew as he watched man and dog at work what was going through his head: you'd think they'd have a machine that could do that, wouldn't you?

Ickornshaw Moor looked as though the sun had never shone on it. It exuded gloom, and the stories of wildcats that once roamed these parts made me keep glancing over my shoulder. I'd been told people still cut peat up here for fuel and I had this fleeting image of walking past peasants with hunchbacks and boils, toiling up to their waists in mud. But the only thing of interest was another piece of ladies' underwear, this time a pair of pale green knickers, tied to a branch of heather. What was the story here? A slip yesterday, knickers today. Were they escaped pieces of washing? Had I stumbled into a lingerie chase? Maybe they belonged to my friends from Liverpool. All this talk of equipment was a front. Underneath their breathable clothing systems they were wearing ladies' underwear.

I reached Cowling. A curtain flicked in a window; a man unloading sand from a pickup nodded at me. Otherwise my passing through this village went unnoticed. But then Cowling didn't look as though it would notice a meteorite land on the green. There would be the same flick of curtains and nod of the head and then it would be back to normal.

Much more attention was paid to me by the herd of cows that came charging across a field that afternoon, as soon as they saw me trying to lift Boogie over the stile. They gathered in an unruly mob below the wall, snorting like dragons, stomping their hooves, demanding I throw him

to them. 'You've got to show them who's boss,' I yelled
at Boogie, struggling to lift him up the steps. 'You've got
to impose yourself on the situation. Dive in there and take
control!'

He slipped out of my grasp and chained himself to a five
bar gate.

I consulted my map. A short detour was possible, and
since the previous night's excursion to Bradford, I had
decided to take every detour and diversion I could. That
seemed to be the way to get the most out of the Pennine
Way. Sure enough, within minutes of coming off the route
I had been invited indoors and was sitting in someone's
centrally heated cottage, being mothered over and fed
refreshments. I sat there thinking: this sort of thing doesn't
happen in England, does it?

Actually it wasn't me who had been invited in so much
as Boogie, by one of those charming elderly women who
can't resist ugly little dogs and seem to think that the reason
they're ugly is because they're being poorly treated and
must be taken inside, sat by the boiler, and given milky
tea in a big bowl with crumbled Digestives in.

'Poor dog,' she said. 'Look at his little furrowed brow.
What he needs is a Lemsip and an electric blanket on
number 4.'

Just the sort of hypochondriac Boogie feels at home
with and likes to encourage with all the dramatic skill
he possesses. As we crossed the threshold, he had put
on his stiff-legged war wound act. 'The poor dog's
injured,' said the woman. 'He shouldn't be walking
the Pennine Way. Are you sure you're feeding him
enough?'

'He eats more than I do.'

'You can afford to lose the weight.'

I took that remark on the chin. Rather like Boogie, I'd
decided that if someone wanted to sit me down in their

kitchen and press Digestives and cups of tea on me, they
could be as rude as they liked.

'He's got a problem with his ankle,' she said, and
examined Boogie as he rolled over and displayed his
wedding tackle. Suddenly she jumped up and went to
the fridge and wrote on a piece of paper the word Leslie,
then sat down again. It was a list of names under the heading
Telephone. In fact there were lists stuck everywhere round
the house. The fridge alone had a shopping list, an odd-job
list, a gardening list, a telephone list, and a miscellaneous
list, all with items ticked or waiting to be ticked. I sat by the
Aga, where neatly arranged tea-towels hung from the rail,
thinking how different homes can be. There was nothing
on any of the surfaces here. Everything had been put away
in marked jars in a cupboard. The biscuits had come out
of a jar with the word biscuit written on it. The tea came
out of a jar marked tea. I made a promise to myself that
if I ever owned a jar marked biscuits I'd put anything in
it other than biscuits.

'Did you hear me?' she said. 'His ankle's poorly.'

'Just a bit stiff,' I answered. 'He's getting fit.'

The warm kitchen and the sound of Radio 2 coming
from another room made me start to feel sleepy. 'Better
go,' I said, and she gave me a piece of cake wrapped in
cling film.

'Thank you very much,' I said. 'You've been very
kind.'

'Give it to him at tea time,' she ordered.

'Right.'

We left and I ate the cake before I was out of sight of
the house.

Lothersdale had a post office shop, and so far between were
these oases I never liked to pass one without going in. They
were such reassuring places. I felt the urge to buy that

jig-saw with the sun-yellowed label, or that tin of carrots, or that 'Happy Birthday to My Grandpa' birthday card, just to chirp the postmistress's spirits up, to let her know that I was on her side, that I too believed supermarkets and out-of-town shopping parks were but a passing trend and soon people would realise their folly and revert to buying their weekly supplies at the village store.

I rummaged through the ice cream cabinet and bought a Magnum ice cream because my wife likes them. To please the postmistress I bought a pie and a slab of cake as well, and when that didn't cheer her up I bought some stamps and postcards. Hers was an original but highly effective sales technique. How refreshing, I thought, as she added up the cost, not to be subjected to name tags and smiles from beaming cashiers.

'Thank you very much,' I said, and when she didn't reply I almost bought a tin of Quality Street.

We sauntered through the afternoon, up to windy Pinhaw Beacon where the view was of hedges, farms and rolling fields. Insects motored around my hat and I could hear the distant hum of tractors. If it hadn't been for some ominous-looking peaks to the north this would all have been more redolent of Sussex than the Pennines.

Having survived the days on the high moorland I deserved to take things easy. I sat under a wall and read three pages of *Wuthering Heights* and felt my eyelids droop again. A glint of metal caught my eye and I saw a 20p. piece stuck upright in a cowpat. The pat was a firm and sticky one, and the coin was jutting out just enough to make it grabbable. I demurred, glanced around me. Maybe I was being filmed on that silly TV programme. Maybe someone was watching me from the bushes, waiting to see how low someone would stoop for a 20p. piece. When I tried to pull it out I'd find it had been cemented in. I left it where it was: I wasn't falling for that.

We came down through farmyards and under old railway lines into Thornton-in-Craven. A van was parked down a side road and the man in the back was sorting through his shelves of videos for hire. Boogie sniffed luxuriously, inhaled the smell of hot dust the way he would a fish supper. Had he been human, I think a video rental business would have been his chosen profession.

I glanced in the van. The collection of videos was large but seemed to consist entirely of copies of *Nightmare on Elm Street* and everything Disney had ever made. I asked the man what were the most popular rentals and he said, 'They like horror round here.'

Here were all these quaint cottages with roses growing up the front, and neat hedges and estate cars parked outside, and at night the residents pulled the curtains and locked the door and sat down to watch vampires being disembowelled.

'It's funny,' went on the video man, ''cos people in towns tend to like comedy romance, *When Harry met Sally*, *Roxanne*, that sort of thing. But out here in the sticks . . . it's horror.'

I asked him what he liked to watch. 'Oh, I like the old black and white stuff. *Casablanca*, best film ever made,' he said, and he shook his head sadly. He'd taken the place of the mobile library; driving round the countryside offering people celluloid thrills, recommending a romance with Greta Garbo or a thriller with Peter Lorre, and all they wanted was a night out with Freddie Kruger.

I'd thought I might stop the night in Thornton but, as with a number of villages we'd passed through, the road which had once brought it life had now overwhelmed it, and traffic roared through ignoring everything but the service station. 'How far is Gargrave?' I asked a man cutting his hedge, and he smacked his lips and said, 'Well it used to be about five miles.'

Such an enigmatic response needed to be acted upon and so I pushed on. But then, some way further, I came across various places that offered accommodation and I decided to stop. I didn't want to walk all evening. I wanted to sit out in a pub garden and inhale the honeysuckle and phone home and tell them what a good time I was having and how all this talk about the Pennine Way being a wet slog was untrue.

'No dogs,' said the woman at a farm when I asked for a bed. She was standing in her kitchen, smoking a cigarette with an inch of ash hanging on the end.

'Not to worry,' I said, relieved that I didn't have to stay there. You could immediately tell what some places were like.

But then she took me by the arm and said, 'On second thoughts he can sleep in the barn, can't he? He'll like that.'

I was about to tell her that Boogie wouldn't like that at all, but then I thought: this is what it's all about, back to basics, in the barn, carousing with all the other farm dogs. This is just what he needs.

The barn was full of farmyard debris, old tractor parts and smashed chicken coops. In one corner was a kennel. 'He'll be fine in that,' said the woman.

Boogie peered inside and smelt the bed of straw; looked at me with an 'imagine having to sleep in that, honestly what some poor dogs have to put up with'; watched me as I put a bowl of complete dog food inside; suspected nothing as he jumped in and stuffed his face; heard the awful clunk of the door closing and the bolt sliding into place; turned round slowly with an 'I don't believe I fell for that, the oldest trick in the book. Come back!'

I was led into the house, up some creaky old stairs. 'You can have young Steven's room,' said the woman. 'He's away the weekend. He won't mind. Breakfast at 8.30. It's a pound extra for the dog. You can pay me now or in a few minutes, whichever suits you.'

The room was dusty and littered with the scraps of young Steven's life. Nothing homey like pictures, just debris blown to all corners: a Dr Who book, some body building magazines, a waste bin with more litter outside it than in, a tin of Whitedent for cleaning false teeth. On the floor by the bed was an alarm clock set at 6.30. In a corner I found a pile of guns and weapons magazines mixed with comic annuals. I peered under the bed and found an aerosol containing something for people who owned shoes that pinched their feet. I read all the directions on the can, wondering if a spray of this stuff would make your shoes bigger or your feet smaller.

A picture of Steven was forming. A young man with dentures who could handle a gun, he got up at 6.30, squeezed into shoes that were too tight for him, then went to work and came home and worked-out, before going to bed and reading Dr Who. I wondered what he did for a living. A pair of cufflinks lay on the dressing table. He was a salesman, I decided. I opened a wardrobe and there was nothing inside but a pool cue. He wasn't a salesman, he was a rookie pool player, waiting for his first big break. That's where he was this weekend of course, playing in a competition somewhere. His tooth had been knocked out by a flying pink.

I opened the window. The room smelt of socks and what was worse was they weren't my socks. In fact the whole house smelt. It had looked beautiful from outside, but within it smelt of damp and old carpets and blocked drains. I sat on the bed awhile and felt annoyed with myself for being so meek, knowing that the only reason places like this got away with it was because people like me put up with it. I wished I was the sort who could just march out.

I went and got Boogie and we walked up to the local
pub, where a party was underway. The function room
had been taken over by a load of men singing loudly and
drinking a lot. One lad came rolling out with a silver jacket
and a thin moustache, looking how I imagined Steven to
look. I asked the barmaid what was going on and she said,
'I don't know. I'm not allowed in there.'

I wandered round the pub looking for someone to talk
to. By the fireplace two men were discussing the lottery.
Someone they knew seemed to have won.

'Lucky bastard. Eight million quid.'

'It'll spoil his life.'

'No it won't.'

'He'll lose all his friends.'

'I'll be his friend.'

'Bollocks!'

I sat at a table opposite a man with a pint pot in one
hand and a book entitled *A Dictionary of Trout Flies* in
the other. I was wondering how to start a conversation
with him, when there was a familiar voice behind me, a
Liverpudlian voice: 'I knew you were staying at the farm.
I said so, didn't I, Tony?'

Good old Tony and Doug. They sat down and squashed
up to the man with the *Dictionary of Trout Flies*.

'You're wondering how we knew you were staying at
the farm, aren't you?' said Doug.

'How?'

'We saw your boots in the hall,' said Tony. 'I said to
Doug, those are that bloke with the dog's boots. The bloke
who's not walking the Pennine Way. Brasher boots.'

The man with the *Dictionary of Trout Flies* was peering
over his book, listening to us. I didn't want to be in
a conversation which someone else was eavesdropping
on. I wanted to be eavesdropping on someone else's
conversation.

'Did you see that piece of ladies' underwear up on Ickornshaw moor?' asked Tony.

'Yes, I did. What do you make of that?'

He shrugged. Doug said, 'I found a pair of fishnet tights once, walking in the Wirral.'

I looked at the man with the *Dictionary of Trout Flies* and he averted his eyes back to the page. He obviously came here every night and hid behind that book, listening to the conversations of Pennine Way walkers.

Doug said, 'It's not very good, is it? The farm.'

'No, it's not,' I said.

'The toilet seat won't stay up,' said Tony.

'No,' said Doug.

'I mean, after a hard day's walking the last thing you want is a toilet seat that won't stay up,' said Tony.

And the man with the *Dictionary of Trout Flies* slammed it shut, got up and left.

'I've got to make a phone call,' I said.

I went to the public phonebox and spent a long time calling home. Catherine said, 'The house is full of old newspapers.'

'That's because I'm not there to clear them up.'

'You clear away the old newspapers?'

'Yes.'

'I never knew that.'

'Whenever I pass through a room I pick up a newspaper and put in on the pile in the garage.'

'All this time and I never knew that.'

It's good to know you're missed, I thought, as I walked back to the farm. When I tried to lead Boogie back into the kennel he protested again: if you think I'm going back in that box while you live it up indoors with a welcoming fruit bowl and herbal shampoos you've got another think coming.

So I threw a packet of peanuts in his bowl and he dived

inside the kennel, then stopped and stared at the ceiling with an 'I don't believe it! I fell for it again!'

I went to my room and got ready for bed, and when I pulled back the sheets I saw they were stained so I got dressed again and marched down to the house to get angry with the woman.

She had that same cigarette, with an inch of ash hanging from it, balanced on her lip. I said, 'Excuse me, I'm sorry to trouble you, I know it's getting late, but . . . you appear to have forgotten to change the sheets.'

'Oh,' she said.

'I mean if you just give me another set I'll do it.'

She gave me another set. I said, 'Thanks, sorry,' and went back upstairs. And the clean ones were as dirty as the dirty ones.

Under the pillow I found a business card, one of Steven's. He wasn't a snooker player. I'd been right first time: he was a salesman, and he sold tractors.

Now we were well into what was known as the Aire Gap, the vale of the River Aire which separates the gritstone of the south from the limestone of the north. It's here that the Pennine Way rubs shoulders with the Leeds-Liverpool canal for just a mile or so, before it bears off to climb up and over a hill and into Gargrave.

But the canal leads to Gargrave as well, it just goes round the hill instead of over it, and I was so enjoying walking by water I decided to stick with the towpath. It was a pleasant change not to have to navigate with maps or look for signposts, but just to follow the bend of the waterway.

It was so quiet that morning, not a breath of wind. The countryside was a still life, not a ripple disturbed the water. Two men stood way across a field and I could hear their voices clearly. I walked through a gate and closed it after me and the clank made magpies rise in a tree a half mile away.

The Leeds-Liverpool was the last of the trans-Pennine canals to be built. Its period of prosperity was brief, but like all of them, it's now resurgent thanks to the popularity of canal boat cruising. I hadn't walked very far before I passed a narrowboat that was just getting underway. The man at the helm asked 'Walking the Pennine Way?' He was wearing a Scoobie-Doo T-shirt.

I replied that I was, and he said, 'My name's Jim. Want a lift to Gargrave?'

Why not? A pleasant cruise on an old narrowboat, feet up, newspaper, cup of tea and be in Gargrave by ten o'clock.

In fact travelling by narrowboat is, I discovered, slower than walking and by the time you've worked a few locks it's a lot more tiring as well.

Unless you're driving of course, like Jim was, in which case you just stand at the back and drink tea, and natter. He was on holiday with his wife. She did all the locks and he did all the steering. She prepared all the food and he did all the eating.

A bowl of cereal appeared with sliced-up strawberries in it, looking just the way it does in the picture on the box. Jim spoke with his mouth full: 'I'd love to do the Pennine Way. It's on my list of ambitions. Is it as tough as everyone says?'

It hadn't really been tough. 'Very tough,' I said

'Do you get depressed?'

Everyone had warned me about getting depressed because I was doing it on my own, but I didn't seem to have spent much time on my own. 'You do get depressed, yes,' I said.

'Why are you doing it?'

'Because I live right at the start,' I said, and for the first time it struck me there might be something more to it than that. Surely I wasn't someone who had always wanted to walk the Pennine Way and was doing it now while he still could?

We chugged along, passing ugly fisherman with rods that stretched right across the canal. Jim said, 'I can't understand those blokes and their big rods. If they want to catch the fish on the other side of the canal, why don't they sit over there?'

He was enjoying himself, winding through the country-side in this groove of water, and when there were no locks it really was the most effortless way to travel. 'It's the perfect holiday,' he said. 'The only trouble with being on a narrowboat is no matter what you do, you end up with a wet bum.'

Mary his wife appeared with tea and Mr Kipling cakes. Everything she passed through the hatch looked like a serving suggestion. 'Elevenses,' she said, although it wasn't yet ten.

Jim smiled lovingly at her. There was nothing these two would have liked more than to sail this narrowboat into a long thin sunset, but they had to be back in Nuneaton on Sunday and in their respective offices on Monday.

Jim said, 'Dog's good company, I bet.'

Boogie had been looking at the floor shaking his head in disgust most of the morning, still not recovered from the ignominy of spending a night behind bars. But now he was on the prow looking smug, largely because he was riding on something rather than walking. I watched him up there, nose in the air, looking superior. He would have made a good barge dog.

We jumped off at Gargrave lock and I stood and waved at Jim and Mary for what felt like ages as they chugged round the bend out of sight. Then I went into the village to buy another bag of complete dog food.

Gargrave had a pleasant position on a curve of the River Aire. It had old bridges and quaint cottages and cafés to sit and write postcards outside. But like Hebden Bridge and Thornton-in-Craven before it, Gargrave was overrun by traffic. There was little peace as trucks and cars and caravans bumped over the old bridges, and the quaint cottages reverberated in shock. And if you sat outside a café writing postcards, as I did, you breathed little but exhaust fumes.

Most of these places had campaigns for bypasses, but more roads would just create more traffic, and you felt it was really time that more drastic measures were taken. It was easy to become sanctimonious as a walker and stride into a village, take one look at it and say cars should be banned and then walk out again, but the sound of slow strangulation by traffic was the lasting impression in all these places. They couldn't survive much more of this hammering, as HGVs forced their way through the narrow streets, clipping off the edges of the buildings. One day one truck too many would trundle through Gargrave and the village would shudder and collapse like a house of cards.

A phone rang in a public phone box. These are irresistible moments. I answered it and a lad said, 'Is there a skinhead waiting in the shelter next door?'

I looked in the shelter, but it was occupied by a couple of women selling jigsaws and old china for charity.

'No,' I said.

'Well, if you see a skinhead walking around, will you tell him to phone me?'

'OK. Phone who?'

'He'll know.' And he hung up.

I went to the supermarket for supplies, keeping an eye out for a skinhead and a postbox. Gargrave has a number of receptacles secured to trees and posts for the disposal of dog poo. Boogie took a look at one and thought: just how the hell am I supposed to get up there? The idea is of course that owners carry shovels around with them and tidily deposit the waste. This is an excellent facility, but they've gone and painted the receptacles red and from a distance they do look like postboxes. I stopped myself in time, but it's a safe bet that a number of postcards of Gargrave have ended up under a pile of doggie-does rather than on Auntie Janet's mantelpiece.

As we walked out of town I did pass a skinhead, or someone with a short haircut anyway, a lapsed skinhead. I said to him, 'I've just had a phone call from someone who wants you to phone him back.'

And the guy looked at me and walked past, giving me a wide berth. And I can't say I blame him.

We headed north on the path to Malham, through creamy pasture. It was Saturday and rambling clubs were out and about. Behind me I could see a group coming down from Eshton Moor. I increased my speed, hoping to outstrip them, but these guys were travelling. They moved down the hillside and over the bridge across the Aire like something military, twenty or so of them, all in brightly coloured breathable clothing.

I decided to stop and let them get ahead. They came along the riverbank at me with heads up, all ready with a nod and a smile and a friendly remark: 'lovely day for it.' 'Dog's enjoying himself.' 'Smashing day for it.' 'Can't you get the dog to carry that pack?'

I said hello and gave a little wave to every one of them, which was ridiculous, and is how hikers get to suffer from repetitive strain injury. Ahead the path was flat and it wound along the river bank into the distance. I didn't want them in front of me all afternoon, so I lay down in the grass and gazed at the sky. It was every shade of grey you could imagine, but all high cloud, no sign of rain. No rain on the Pennine Way for a week now – it was unheard off. I wasn't complaining, but why wouldn't it rain on me? This was more than good luck. This was weird. A drop here or there would have been reassuring. Again I had the feeling I was doing something wrong.

A woman came sauntering down the bank. She stopped when she saw me and asked if a group of hikers had gone by.

I said it had, and she shook her head. 'They go far too fast, they don't see anything. I normally walk with my friend Michele but she's got food poisoning.'

She had her OS map open, and as the breeze picked it up it flapped out of control. She struggled to fold it, then handed it to me and said, 'Would you fold my map for me?'

'I . . . sure.'

'Someone told me recently that men's spacial ability is better than women's.'

'What?'

'Men can fold a map, whereas women can fold a table cloth. Tests have proved it.'

I tried to fold her map but got myself in a complete tangle, putting creases in all the wrong places. She snatched it back with a 'just as I thought!', and marched off to catch up the group she was walking with instead of Michele.

I threw stones in the river in the hope Boogie would dive in after them and wash off the cow dung he'd rolled in. The plan didn't work, of course, and it ended up a hands-on job. I took my boots off and waded in and a wrestling match began. Twenty minutes later the dung was off Boogie and all over me.

We followed the Aire upstream, through flowery meadows. The cattle were after us again. In one field they were in the far corner as I threw Boogie down from the stile. I saw them look up and come cantering across to head us off, but I judged that, if we hurried, we could make it to the stile on the other side of the field before they reached us. I set off running as fast as was possible with a pack on my back, and urged Boogie to follow.

Then when I got to the other side I couldn't find the stile into the next field. I ran frantically up and down the hedge while the stampede came straight for us. Then there it was, and of course it had to be one of those ladder stiles that meant I would have to stop and take off my pack and lift Boogie up onto the platform on the top, and then climb over and help him down. I turned and resigned myself to being trampled. Boogie however took one look at the oncoming cattle and sprinted to the stile, crouched, leapt and sailed over it like a steeplechaser. I watched dumbfounded. I turned to the cattle and they had stopped and were looking dumbfounded themselves. I climbed the stile and looked down at Boogie who was sitting on the other side licking his balls.

'You've been able to do that all along, haven't you?'

He tried to look embarrassed. I tried to look angry. It could well have been the moment of bonding I was seeking.

We walked along the banks of the Aire all afternoon, a charming and easy walk, full of bird life and through more of these glorious meadows.

I called in on the village of Aireton, walked once around it and then sat down on the green and watched a woman walk from room to room in a house opposite that had no curtains.

Presently a man and his dog sat next to me and said: 'treacle toffee?' and he offered me a crumpled bag. I took one and immediately my mouth was clamped. 'Where are you walking to?' he asked.

'The Pnnne Wyy,' I mumbled.

'Where?'

'Pnnne Wwy.'

'Where?'

I showed him my guide book. He nodded. Then he
looked at Boogie and asked, 'He's not a guide dog or
anything, is he?'

I shook my head.

'I met a bloke once before, walking the Pennine Way
with a guide dog. The animal looked annoyed, you know.
Well it's asking too much of a guide dog that is. I mean,
down the shops, round the park, to the library, that's all
right. But the Pennine Way? That's above and beyond.'

We strode on past a fine old mill and then the river
sharply narrowed and disappeared into a hole in the ground,
as if hiding its head under the covers, as if it knew what was
coming.

Now the land ahead began to rise into cliffs and all the
hills beyond were steep and rimmed with silver outcrops.
We were entering limestone country and everything was
about to change.

4. A Dingo in the Dales

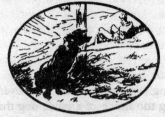

'The mountains and the hills will break into song,' proclaimed the poster outside the Methodist Chapel in Malham.

'Not if I have anything to do with it they won't,' muttered a man licking an ice cream, and he elbowed his wife until she laughed.

But if anywhere along the Pennine Way were likely to break into song, then Malham was the spot. The whole place was a performance. Geological drama leapt out at you from round every corner; limestone cliff to the left, spectacular waterfall to the right, displays that made your jaw drop. It had the feel of a theme village, as if all things geologically impressive had been bought, uprooted and re-erected on this site.

There was a good audience here as well. All paths led to Malham, and it had international appeal. German kids were yelling in the camp site. Japanese families rode round on bicycles. Scandinavians loafed around the bunk houses. Americans with big rucksacks knocked over souvenirs in the gift shop.

I went for a stroll that evening with my hands in my pockets along Gordale Beck over another carpet of wildflowers ('Single file through the meadows, please', asked the sign). We reached a perfect waterfall at Janet's Foss and should really have turned round there and gone back for haddock and chips in the pub, but then ahead of us was this splendid cliff with a violent gash in its face, and before I knew it I was climbing a rockfall and my pulse was thumping.

The gash was a ravine called Gordale Scar and at first it appeared impenetrable, but a path followed the river bed, sneaking round corners, piercing the heart of the cleft. Soon we found ourselves standing at the bottom of an open-topped cylinder of rock, and in front of us the unmistakable sight of two Australians sitting on rocks drinking beer in the sunset.

'Beautiful, eh?' I said.

'Absolutely. We just had to stop and have one of these.'

'Yeah,' said his mate.

'Is there a way through to the cliff top,' I asked. I wanted to climb up and come back to the village via the ridge.

'It's a scramble,' said one. 'But you can do it.'

I started up. The other lad called after me, 'Don't get excited, there's no pub at the top.'

I wondered if Boogie could make it. I knew he didn't want to. I knew he would rather have gone back to Malham and toured the dustbins for the *Good Dustbin Guide to Great Britain* that he was compiling. But I thought, if he could climb ladder stiles he could climb the Matterhorn, and with a push here and a shove there he was able to clamber up the downfall deeper into the ravine. An evil-eyed limestone sculpture presented itself, a ring of rock like an eye socket, with water pouring through. I was passing through a limestone version of Hades.

We kept climbing towards the sky, with the view and the drop opening out below us. The sound of rushing water diminished and then we were at the rim. I stuck my head over, to be confronted face to face with a sheep.

I made a noise that sounded like some comic book

'*Arrgh*!' and almost sprang back, a dumb thing to do when you've just reached a cliff top, but I'd rarely seen a sheep at such close quarters. This one had a superbly dumb expression that was only good at giving double-takes, and a wonderfully vacant look that said, 'hang on a minute!' It looked as if it had observed Boogie and me and had sent the information back to its brain and was in the process of waiting for a response to determine what action to take. Finally the command came back to run like crazy, and the animal took off on its fragile legs.

Up here were broad swards of emerald pasture with limestone puncturing the surface like a skin disease. The sky was grey marbled with maroon, and these colours created a moodiness. Sunshine and blue skies would have given a chocolate box dazzle, would have recreated the postcards, which didn't do it justice.

I followed a footpath, hoping it would lead back down to the village, but then suddenly we were standing on top of the bone-like limestone pavement that caps the cliff above Malham Cove. The ground gave way and we were left there, above the birds, looking down on the huge panorama of the Aire valley and all the country we'd covered over the last two days.

The cove is a hugely impressive limestone amphitheatre, and its accessibility from Malham village means that a constant stream of visitors make the effort to walk the dressed path, take a snap and go back to the car. This has resulted in considerable erosion, but you can't spoil something as grand as this, not without explosives. The cliff dwarfs all human activity. Only the swallows and jackdaws that swoop in and out of its crevices seem to have truly conquered it.

We climbed down the staircase to the river that emerges from the base of the cliff. On the path back to the village along the bank, I was the only one who wasn't walking arm in arm with a lover. I wasn't going to whisper sweet nothings into Boogie's ear, and so I phoned home when I got back to the village.

Francis answered. 'It's me,' I said.

'Who?'

'Your dad.'

'How's Boogie?'

Outside, walking across the village square, I could see the lads from Liverpool. They saw me in the phonebox and waved. Catherine came on. I told her how much I missed her, how sensational Gordale Scar was and how we must all come back here one day. . . .

There was a rap on the window and a yell. 'We're going to the pub,' and there was Doug's nose pressed against the glass. 'Oh sorry, you're on the phone.'

Catherine said, 'I'm glad you called. I can't find the dustbags for the vacuum cleaner.'

There were two pubs in the village. I tried to think which one would appeal to Doug and Tony and then went into the other one, and of course there they were in the corner drinking Guinness. 'Are you sure you're not walking the Pennine Way?' asked Tony.

'No, no,' I insisted, but when I went to the bar I thought: this is no way to behave towards two fellow Pennine Way walkers. If you're going to be meeting these two every night then it's rude to avoid them. Instead try to enjoy their company.

'Actually I *am* walking the Pennine Way,' I said to them when I sat down.

They looked at me for a moment. Then Doug said, 'You're just saying that.'

'No, really I am.'

'Don't believe you,' said Tony.

'I am, honestly.'

'Pull the other one,' said Doug.

I went to order fish and chips at the food counter. A man asked the barmaid if he could have some cutlery for his meal and she sighed and flung some irons at him. 'Thank you very much,' he said, and she looked at me and muttered, 'Customers!'

Back at the table Tony said, 'Do you like Wainwright?'

Alfred Wainwright, the godfather of ramblers, the man with ever such neat handwriting. Whenever I picture Alfred Wainwright he's in a little house with everything perfectly tidy, with his spice rack in alphabetical order and his shirts filed away according to colour, dark on the bottom getting lighter as they go up, cricket shirts on the top.

'Yes,' I said. 'I like Wainwright.'

Some people thought his books were so precise they took the sense of discovery out of a walk. There was a certain amount of truth in this, but they were all works of love, and he had a good sense of humour. He had the north country in his bones.

'Doug can't stand the bloke,' said Tony.

'Can't stand him,' said Doug.

Doug was an iconoclast. First Gore-tex and now Wainwright.

'I reckon he's good value,' said Tony.

'An impossible man to live with, I wouldn't mind betting,' said Doug. 'He did all those walks on his own, you know, and I reckon that was 'cos no-one would go with him.'

Tony threw his eyes up at the ceiling. Clearly Doug made a habit of badmouthing Wainwright. In fact Doug was talking in the tones of a man who had a grudge. Maybe Wainwright had run off with his wife.

I said, 'Do you two get on all right?'

They had never expected such a question. They avoided eye contact.

'I mean, it's not easy being in someone's company all day long. It's a lot to ask for two people to walk together for three weeks. It's not like spending twenty minutes of your lunchbreak with each other, is it?'

Tony was looking at Doug but Doug wasn't looking at Tony.

I went on, 'It can put a strain on any relationship if you're not used to it. Sometimes I get pissed off with my dog and sometimes he gets pissed off with me. Don't you, Boogie? Boogie!'

I nudged Boogie and he ignored me.

'See, he's pissed off with me now.'

'We get on fine, don't we Doug?' said Tony.

'We're mates,' said Doug.

There was a silence. I ate my meal.

Tony smacked his lips. Doug looked out of the window. I opened my mouth to make an observation about carrots and how everywhere I'd eaten on this walk, carrots had been compulsory and every pub seemed to cook them to a pulp, but as usual Doug started to say something at the same time.

'After you,' said Doug

'No, no after you,' I insisted.

'I was just wondering if you had negative equity?' said Doug.

The man from the Malham sweet shop opened up and surveyed the day with the smile he reserved for Sunday mornings. Then he dragged out a four foot high cardboard cut-out ice cream cone, which he stood on the pavement, and which fell over as soon as he went back inside.

Boogie was limping again, the way he did now whenever we walked through a village, hoping someone would take pity and invite him indoors for a bit of pampering. I wasn't feeling so good myself. I'd spent the evening talking to some tall, thin Scandinavian youths about the things they did in their long dark winters above the Arctic Circle.

'It is a time for reflection,' said one.

'I go to the cinema,' said another.

'I play underwater rugby,' said a third, and when I showed an interest, he talked long and seriously about the many pleasurable weekends he'd spent the previous winter, scrummaging for a water-filled ball at the bottom of a swimming pool in Tromso.

They probably stayed up like that every night, but late nights were the one thing I couldn't cope with on this trip. I'd woken early as usual, and hadn't been able to sleep any longer, so I had got going. Now already I was feeling weary. I felt like I'd been walking for weeks, and yet, as I studied my maps over breakfast, I saw I'd barely covered a quarter of the distance to Scotland.

But distance wasn't the priority here, I reminded myself. Today, particularly, was a day to take slowly, a day to savour. From Malham the Pennine Way takes the walker through the best of the Yorkshire Dales' limestone country, and I was fully expecting the next fifteen miles to be some of the most memorable of the entire route.

We climbed up to the top of the Cove again. There was the echo of a cathedral about it on this Sunday morning, and the rambling groups were abroad in numbers paying their respects. They appeared whenever you positioned yourself behind a rock and unzipped your fly, and as the morning went on they became so numerous I felt as if I was caught in a sort of diaspora heading north to some promised land. It's tempting in situations like this to look at the crowds and think how the countryside has been spoiled irrevocably by paths like the Pennine Way. The alternative is to think how fine it is to see people taking advantage of the access to the land that now exists, and that erosion is the price you have to pay for this. I'm sure Tom

Stephenson would have subscribed to the latter view. My only complaint was the insistence all these ramblers had of saying hello to every other rambler, and expecting them to say hello in return. In Malham this is a bit like saying hello to everyone as you walk down Fifth Avenue. If you are in a group, you can get away with just a nod, and someone else can do the hello, but if you're on your own, you end up saying 'hello!' until your tongue is in a knot. As I headed towards Malham Tarn a group of about fifteen walkers approached, and I decided that this had all got out of hand, and I would say 'hello' to the first one, 'hello' to number eight and 'hello' to number thirteen. Three 'hellos', one per five walkers. That was good enough.

No it wasn't. Anyone I didn't reply to slowed and gave me a blazing look, making it clear they weren't going to pass until I responded with some greeting. If I still resisted, their faces crumpled and they looked suicidal, as if I'd singled them out to be rude to, as if they'd only come out of the house that morning to say 'hello' to someone, and now they'd been ignored their day was ruined. I tried avoiding eye contact but it did no good; they just shouted at me until I paid attention. By the time I had passed them all, the word 'hello' had no meaning any more. It was just a sound.

For some reason, though, you don't have to say 'hello' to ramblers if you are overtaking them. No-one expected you to turn round and smile and greet them as you passed. This was a relief because I was gaining on a large group for about a mile up the Dry Valley above Malham Cove. I began to overtake them one by one.

'I'm not going to marry him until he pulls his socks up and that's all there is to it. I've had enough.'

'It's a drop in salary but the potential of the company is huge.'

'Did you watch *One Foot in the Grave* the other night? It reminded me of you.'

As I was halfway through the crowd, a drizzle started. They walked on regardless until the leader stopped without warning, almost causing a pile-up behind him, and pulled out his waterproofs. Every member of the group did the same. I decided to get past them all and then put mine on without stopping, so that I could pull ahead. But then of course as soon as I pulled my jacket out and shook it at the clouds, the rain stopped, and I looked behind me to see the ramblers were all bumping into each other again as they halted to remove their waterproofs. Ahead lay a piece of woodland, the only cover in this exposed landscape. I headed into it and never looked back.

We had reached Malham Tarn, which looked bitterly cold and unappealing, although when Charles Kingsley had stayed at Malham Tarn House, he had been inspired enough to create *The Water Babies*. Now the house and the surrounding woods are a Field Studies Centre, and the smell of home cooking rises in steam from the buildings. Everyone I saw in the grounds was looking carefully at the earth or studying the sky through binoculars. They were all so friendly.

'What are you looking for?' I asked a young woman. 'Snails,' she said with a lovely smile, and wiped the hair out of her eyes with her mucky fingernails.

Fountains Fell loomed ahead, looking like a morning's hard work. It was a sprawling hill and the path staggered from side to side as it climbed. We suffered a number of false summits, but when we reached the top the climax was huge: a stunning view of Penyghent hit us full in the face.

It made you want to stop and say something out loud, like 'wow!' or 'strewth!', to the nearest living thing. In my case that was Boogie, but he was looking the other way, nose tuned to a far-off bacon sandwich.

In fact the sandwich wasn't as far off as I thought. It

belonged to the big man and his little dog sitting behind a wall having lunch. Boogie trotted over and gave them a look of such desperation it could only say: you can sleep with me if you give me a bite of that.

I called to the man, 'Some view!' And as luck would have it, he knew all the peaks in the panorama and, very gracefully for a man of his size, he gave a 180-degrees flourish and named every one of them.

'That one's Whernside, that one's Penyghent, that one is called Ingleborough. . . .' and at that point he filled his mouth with sandwich and I didn't catch the rest, only, 'and my dog here is called Bronson,' before he sat down again.

Not that names were important at a moment like this. These hills were huge and still and filled your vision, great animals that had slept and slept for millions of years. Penyghent was shaped like an anvil. Whernside, behind it, was a hulk with a stairway of summits. Ingleborough looked a prone animal.

These three comprised The Three Peaks, and climbed together they made up the twenty-mile Three Peaks Challenge. You can complete this walking, jogging, on a bicycle or walking backwards holding your breath and wearing an arrow-through-the-head kit. It doesn't matter, you'll always find someone who has done it faster. 'Someone ran the Three Peaks in three hours,' said my friend with the picnic.

A statistic like that can be depressing when you're taking the whole day to walk the fourteen miles from Malham to Horton-in-Ribblesdale. Especially now that we were going down, down, down, and losing all the precious height we had gained, so that the climb up Penyghent ahead of us looked tougher by the minute. By the time we reached the valley bottom it appeared insurmountable.

This was largely because there didn't seem to be any

route up it. The best way to tackle it, I decided, was not to look. I just stared at my feet, followed the trail and contemplated my future. I thought how this walk was going to change me. 'I'm going to get a rowing machine when I get back,' I promised myself halfway up the slope. 'I'm going to stay fit. And I'm going to handle money better. I'm going to save and buy myself a Triumph. I'm going to dress snappier too. I'm not going to shout at the kids any more. And I'm going to decorate the kitchen, I really am.'

Three quarters of the way up the hill, 'I'm going to start meditating when I get home, you know,' I said to Boogie. 'And I'm going to learn a language at evening class. Languages are important,' and he gave me his 'do what you bleedin' well like mate' face.

The ascent took me the best part of an hour. Then I looked up and saw I was scrambling towards the summit. One last push: 'when I get home I'm going to watch more documentaries and even start flossing my teeth,' I said out loud and looked up to see I'd reached the top. And there, sitting underneath a wall and sheltering from the wind, was the Doncaster Rambling Club, passing round biscuits and having tea from flasks.

'Lovely day for it,' I said, and they ignored me to a member.

We glided down the hill towards Horton-in-Ribblesdale, a refreshing wind in our faces. The trouble with life is that by the time you've had a session on your rowing machine, meditated for the regulation twenty minutes, then been to the college for your Spanish class, and then practised your clarinet, and finally sorted out your bank account, there's no time left to sleep, let alone floss your teeth or paint the kitchen. And shouting at the kids meant you weren't ignoring them.

The view had changed now to take in a large quarry

that looked like a wedding cake layered into the hillside.
Nothing pleasant to look at, but a reminder that quarries
are an industry as old and as much a part of this landscape
and the local economy as farming.

The real action in these parts though is below the surface
rather than on the top. For this is cave country. As you
descend Penyghent, beneath you is a limestone honeycomb
of potholes and passages that surface on these slopes in a
series of openings resembling wounds.

The first you pass on the Pennine Way is Hunt Pot,
which looks like an outsized limestone letterbox. The
second, Hull Pot, is a dirty great hole if ever there was
one, in fact if you're into holes then this is the place
to come, because this is the biggest, dirtiest and greatest
natural hole in England. You're walking along a soft green
path and then suddenly there it is, a hundred metres long
by twenty wide, looking like a blowhole, or some sort of
orifice anyway, belonging to the body of Penyghent.

I stood and gawked, and gawked some more. Presented
with a big hole in the ground it quickly becomes evident
that there is little else to do with it other than stand
and gawk. I glanced around the rim and there were
two other walkers standing and gawking. Three walkers
and one dog gawking at a hole in Yorkshire. It's a funny
old world.

'We saw a hole like this in Norway, didn't we, Gwen?'
said one of the walkers to his partner. They were Australian
and on a whistlestop tour of Europe.

'I don't remember,' said Gwen.

'Yes you do. It was a great pit in the ground surrounded
by hills like this.'

'I mean I don't remember Norway,' said Gwen.

They walked with me down into Horton-in-Ribblesdale,
along a fine grassy lane bordered by walls. It was one of
the many green roads in this area, old trails that undulate

through the hills, firm and true and just asking to be walked on.

'What sort of dog is that, anyway?' asked Gwen.

'He's a cross between a mongrel and something,' I answered.

'Reminds me of a dingo. A dingo in the Dales.'

A team of mountain bikers came flying down the track in flashes of pink and yellow fluorescence, shrieking in delight. They passed with a wave and yell as they flung their bikes into every available puddle and splashed us freely with mud.

'Tenacious animal, the dingo,' said Gwen's man, in Boogie's defence. 'The Wild Dog Destruction Board had to build a 5000-mile fence to keep the dingoes out in Australia.'

Now motorcross bikes were buzzing up the lane, spraying more muck. Sunday was the most restless, unpeaceful day of the week round here.

Gwen sighed and said, 'I love England.'

There was a café in Horton-in-Ribblesdale. I'd not realised how chilly the day had become until I plunged headlong into the fug, and I quickly felt heady amid the thick smell of buns and chips.

Hikers were sitting here with their noses running, clutching mugs and gazing blankly at the steamed up windows. The forlorn face of Boogie gazed back at them, a victim of the No Dogs Allowed rule. He was sitting in the porch tied to an ice cream advert with his eyeballs swinging in the bottom of his eyes as he looked balefully at all customers hoping for a slice of bread pudding, a crust from that fried egg sandwich, the privilege of licking that empty plate of beans on toast.

'Would you like a biscuit, little doggie?' asked a young girl sitting by the window, and she held up her Wagon

Wheel to Boogie who was trying to eat it through
the glass.

'Don't be ·mean,' said her mother, 'or you'll go and
give it him.' She scowled at her daughter and went back
to studying her map of the Yorkshire Moors, which was
odd since this was the heart of the Dales and the Yorkshire
Moors were fifty miles to the east.

The people who ran the café were very helpful. I made a
remark to one of them about the relationship between the
National Park and the local quarry, and before I knew it,
he had launched into an invective aimed at the planning
authorities who, he claimed, were trying to turn the
Dales into a museum and had little or no thought for
local people. Why on earth they insisted on new houses
having tiny windows just to conform to the style of the
older buildings – which had them simply to keep the cold
out – he couldn't fathom. 'We have central heating up
here now, you know.'

I flicked through the pages of the Pennine Way walkers'
log book kept in the café. The man with the rottweiler had
been through ahead of me. And there was that man who
looked like Little John whom I'd met on the first day. This
collection of names went back years, and made me feel
part of a very big club. It was the definitive book on the
Pennine Way, with contributions from walkers worldwide,
each summing up their journey in a sentence, each showing
undying determination to enjoy themselves in adversity,
each ending with an exclamation mark of enthusiasm!

'Rather chilly for June. But can't complain!'

'Wet wet wet, but enjoying it!'

'It's freezing. Ice, snow, wet, zero visibility – great
fun!'

I found only one equivocal entry: 'If anyone catches up
with someone called Lorne. Nobble him for me.'

As I flicked through I tried to think of the worst thing

that had happened to me. I wanted to write something like: 'lost my girlfriend in swamp on Black Hill, but otherwise had wonderful time!' But the worst I could come up with was that I'd had a bad dream in Haworth. I felt embarrassed. I could hardly write 'Edale to Horton and I haven't worn my waterproofs once!' That was just asking for trouble. A flood would wash away the café as I dotted my exclamation mark.

That night I lay in a draughty bunkhouse below a man from Birkenhead who talked in his sleep.

'Place it in the top of the oven on gas mark three for forty minutes,' he mumbled.

I tossed and turned. I was feeling nervous. It had occurred to me I was being treated gently because the gods of the Pennine Way had something truly dreadful in store for me. I was being let off the driving rain and the bogs and the blisters and general misery because very shortly I was going to get hit by lightning. Either that or one of those RAF jets that practised low flying manoeuvres all over the Dales would crashland, and although the plane would miss me, the ejected pilot would land on my back and break my collar bone in three places.

'I only bought it on Monday and it's got a flat battery already,' complained the man from Birkenhead.

I was woken next morning by a goods train rumbling past on the Settle to Carlisle line. And later, as I climbed up into the hills again along another beautiful green road, the railway line was always in view, winding through the wide valley of the Ribble. It was a comforting sight, with the clouds flying overhead, throwing it into light then shadow. Its reputation as the most scenic line in England made it all the more appealing.

It was a bad idea to spend too long gazing into the distance around here though. This was still cave country;

you were never far from an openmouthed pit. Sell Gills
Holes opened on each side of the path, turning the Pennine
Way into a natural bridge. A little further on, Jackdaw Hole
was another knife-wound in the ground. Then at Calf
Holes, cavers, heavily equipped with beards and hat-lights,
were surfacing from the darkness. They looked as if they'd
just seen something that human beings shouldn't see.

There was one cave just off the path called Browgill
Cave, which I'd been told walkers could enter and venture
into for a hundred yards or so. I peered in and shone my
torch into the yawning hole. Boogie had more sense and
sat outside snapping at butterflies as I began to feel my way
carefully down the wet walls.

It was like walking down a throat. Ahead was a blackness,
and water dripped from every crack. I heard voices behind
me and looked back to the mouth of the cave to see some
cavers with all the right equipment entering the hole. I
stood back and let them pass, and asked them where the
cave led. 'We're about to find out,' said the one with the
biggest beard. They wore wet suits and Wellingtons and I
felt so ill-equipped I retreated.

We reached the gorge of Ling Gill, a deep ravine with
sheer sides that made it inaccessible to stock. Left ungrazed
in this way it had maintained its woodland – ash, cherry
and rowan – and was a brief and sylvan glimpse of what
this terrain might have looked like had sheep not been
introduced.

The peace was shattered as another swarm of motorcycle
scramblers passed. I could hear them for a mile or so before
they breached the brow of the hill, and came bumping
along the track in clouds of exhaust. I grabbed hold of
Boogie. It would have been an unfair death for him, to
have survived the streets of London for five years, only
to be run over walking the Pennine Way. The bikes
spluttered off round the bend but you could hear them

for a long time afterwards. They were about as much in tune with the countryside as the RAF jets.

Now the Ribblehead Viaduct that carries the Settle-Carlisle line had come into view, a long and graceful string of 24 arches. I couldn't resist it and I came off the main path and headed down into the valley for a closer look.

A mobile snack-bar was parked near the viaduct. I asked the woman when the next train was due. 'You just missed it,' she said. So I went down to the arches and stood beneath them, getting dripped on. Maybe if I put my ear to the stone I could hear a train coming.

I decided to wait for one. And you can wait a long time for a train on the Settle-Carlisle line. I sat and gazed at the viaduct from Soldiers' Moss where the army of builders' navvies were camped for years during the construction. No doubt when it opened it was regarded as an eyesore, but now it graced the landscape, in the way only railway architecture can.

It got to lunchtime. I was of half a mind to go back to the snack bar and get something to eat, but I knew that as soon as I did, a train would come. A man with a video camera appeared. We both said, 'Do you know when the next train is?'

He announced he was from Norfolk. 'People come to Norfolk for their holidays, but I can never understand it. I'd much rather come here.'

'I went to Norfolk for my holidays once,' I told him.

'See what I mean.'

The clouds danced across the fells making shapes like boats, then castles, then silhouettes of royalty. I was sitting on a rise, gazing at clouds, waiting for a train that was coming I knew not when. I hadn't felt so successful for years.

The man from Norfolk put his camera up to his eye to film the viaduct and I moved out of the way, but he waved me back. 'No, stay where you are,' he said. 'It gives it life. Maybe if you stood up and gazed into the distance.'

So I stood up, suddenly feeling clumsy, running my fingers through my hair, not knowing where to put my hands, first folding them, then stuffing them casually in my pockets, then clutching my chin. I was going to be appearing in this man's living room as he showed his friends and neighbours back in Norfolk the film of his trip to The Dales, and they'd say, 'Who's that bloke who doesn't know what to do with his hands?'

'So you and your dog are walking the Pennine Way?' he said, still filming.

'That's right,'

'What's it like?'

He was interviewing me for his holiday video! He zoomed in on me as I began to mumble, 'Well, it's tough in places but it's very beautiful and I've been very lucky with the weather. Um. . . .'

'And the dog?'

'What about him?'

'Is he enjoying it?'

'I don't know. Yes. He's loving it.'

He put the camera down. 'Does he fetch sticks, your dog?'

'No.'

'I bet he does. Throw one for him; it looks great on the video.'

He passed me a stick. I said, 'You don't understand. The only command this dog knows is: "lie down in front of the fire and eat this crumpet."'

'Go on, throw it!'

I threw it, and Boogie waited until the camera was rolling before he raced after the stick, picked it up on the turn and raced back with it, depositing at the feet of the man from Norfolk. I was stunned. I tried to think of the last time he had fetched something, and I realised he had never fetched anything.

'I didn't quite get that, can he do it again?' asked the man.

And I threw the stick and Boogie ran off with a flourish and did it all again.

'You big tart,' I said to him as we walked up to Ribblehead station. 'Some people will do anything to get on TV.'

We got to the platform and I studied the timetable. As I was standing there a two carriage train chugged round the bend and came to a halt, and a door hissed open right in front of me. I thought: if a train stops when you're standing on a station on the Settle–Carlisle line, then you'd be a fool not to get on it.

There were only about ten people on board. The viaduct seemed an incredible effort of engineering just to get us across this quarter mile dip in the terrain. As we rolled slowly over the first arch the conductor came and stood over me and said, 'Yes?'

'Hang on,' I said. 'This is the best bit. I want to see.'

'It's much better to be on the ground watching the train go over, like that bloke with the video camera down there, look.'

He was right of course, but now I was on the thing I had to go somewhere.

'Where's nice?' I asked.

'Appleby, a couple of stops up the line. The horse fair is on.' He handed me a ticket. 'You'll enjoy Appleby. I went once and saw this horse kick hell out of a brand new Ford Sierra. I'll never go again.'

I quite liked the idea of a horse kicking hell out of a Ford Sierra, and the Appleby Horse Fair was something I'd always wanted to see. This is the kind of luck that happens to some people all the time, I told myself, as I settled into my seat, and now it was happening to me. 'Just watch your pockets,' said the conductor.

It felt strange to be riding on a train. If having nothing to do all day but walk made me feel guilty, the idea of riding when I should have been walking made me feel condemned. But it was a beautiful ride. From Ribblehead the two carriages hauled their way up to Dent through long tunnels and over more fine viaducts. We travelled through tight hills, dotted with white farmhouses that looked very remote. This was the sort of country I imagined W.H. Auden's The Night Mail passing through: 'In the farms as she passes no-one wakes, but a jug in a bedroom gently shakes.'

In winter they used to have snow gangs on this line. In the terrible storms of 1947 it closed for two months. Now the hills were lit with sunshine, but even on a train I had this feeling again that we were tip-toeing across something very fierce.

A man was sitting opposite covered in railway badges. He smiled at me, or at least I thought he was smiling at me, but he was just smiling generally, smiling at everything and everyone. He was a happy man because he was a railway buff and he was on the Settle-Carlisle line, and what was more now he had someone to speak to. As we reached Aisgill he said, '1169 feet. That's the height we're at now. The summit of the line,' and he folded his arms and looked pleased with himself. 'Are you a member of the Friends of the Settle-Carlisle Line?' he asked.

'No. I'm not.'

'I thought you were a member. I thought I'd seen you at the meetings. You look like a member.'

I've been told I resemble many things but never a member of the Friends of the Settle-Carlisle Line.

'It's easy to join,' he said. 'Individual membership seven pounds. Family membership, eight pounds. We were formed back in 1981 when the line was under threat of closure. We put together a rescue package. We saved the Ribblehead Viaduct.'

'Well done,' I said.

He gave me a commentary on the line. There was the junction with the Wensleydale Railway, now closed. There was Kirkby Stephen with its parish church known as the Cathedral of the Dales. And did I know that there was an appeal under way to raise enough money to reinstate a swan-necked water column at Garsdale?

I asked him what he would do if he won the lottery, expecting him to say he'd donate it all to the restoration of the waiting room at Settle Station or something. But I was quite wrong. He said, 'I'd have a cruise round the Caribbean and then buy a big house in the south of France.'

Good for him.

As the train pulled into Appleby there was nothing immediately to suggest the town was gripped with horse fever, but as I walked from the station past semi-detached houses with neat gardens and washed cars, a sweet and sickly smell grew stronger and then sat heavily in the back of the throat. There was a taste of horses, dung and sweat in the air, and in the distance was the scream of police sirens.

Appleby Horse Fair – or New Fair as it is locally known – is a gypsy event, held by Royal Charter since 1685. Once a year they gather here and a barely controlled mayhem grips the town as horses are bought and sold and raced through the streets.

As I turned onto the embankment along the river Eden, the road was lined with dark-eyed, brightly-dressed people, drinking heavily, laughing uproariously, and side-stepping the piles of horse shit everywhere. Horses were tied to anything that didn't move. People were up lampposts and lying in the street. It was a scene out of the wild west.

'Watch your back,' yelled someone and grabbed my arm as a horse and buggy appeared over the brow of the hill, galloping for all its worth on tarmac that made it slip and slide. It was being whipped and yelled at by a teenage driver who sat with his legs in the air and his eyes shut. The police tried to slow him down but they were powerless 'What are they going to do?' said one man with a knot of ear-rings. 'Take his number?'

Boogie and I pushed our way through the crowd and the debris, Boogie operating like a Hoover as he trawled the pavements, picking up hotdogs, fish and chips, ice creams. He was in a feeding frenzy.

We made it down to the river and watched the horses being washed. This was the excuse the riders had for bringing their animals into town. They led them into the stream and threw buckets of water over them, making them steam, and the spectacle drew a big crowd watching from the banks and the bridge. A man with a flashing gold tooth eyed me and limped over. His breath was a blast of alcohol as he said, 'Do you want to sell your dog?'

'No. Well . . . how much?'

'I'll give you a table and six dining chairs for him.'

There was a lawlessness about Appleby which I'd never experienced in a town in England before. There were eight-year-olds on horses galloping down the street. The pubs were bursting, full of people shouting with their fingers in someone's face. I heard that in one a billiard table light had been stolen while the landlord was getting something from the top shelf.

The locals were all quoted in the press as being outraged by the whole affair. It was said they either went away or locked their doors for the week. In reality they seemed to have cottoned on. Some were at the bottom of their driveways selling ice cream for a lot of money. It seemed that for all the intrusion, Appleby could cope with this once a year.

And then disaster. One of the horsemen brought his horse into the river without unharnessing the buggy; he just drove the animal and wagon straight into the water. Everyone laughed when the buggy went over and he went flying, but then the horse went over too, and, with the buggy still strapped to it, it couldn't stand up. It lay there struggling while the crowd yelled at the driver to do something. He tried to unbuckle the harness; other riders tried to help him, but by that time the horse was in convulsions, and it drowned right there under the town bridge in front of a thousand people.

There was a hush. Someone pushed me in the back.

'Mother of God,' said a woman, and then shoved her way to the front of the crowd and took out a video camera. It only needed the one, and everyone was taking out cameras. The crowd edged closer to get a better look at the dead beast.

No-one knew what to do. A police siren wailed; a panda car screeched to a halt and the owner of the horse was taken away to be questioned. Eventually a truck with a winch turned up. Two men jumped out and stripped to the waist, and the corpse was hauled out of the river and hoisted into the air. It dripped blood through its nose and the children who had gathered as close as they could squealed and ran away. Then it was dumped in the truck with a thump and driven off, and everyone put their cameras back in their bags. 'The fair's not as exciting as it used to be,' said one man as he turned away.

I walked out of town under the bypass to the encampment where the gypsy caravans were installed in three huge fields.

Here were horse vans and trailers, caravans and sideshows as far as you could see.

'They've been arriving for the last three months,' said a man selling hotdogs. 'And it takes another three for 'em to pack up and leave again.'

I wandered round the stalls. Everywhere deals were being done. In cabals men with hats and bulging pockets talked in thick accents and prodded each other's horses.

But it wasn't just horses for sale. You could buy anything here from garden furniture to jewellery that you knew was real but if it was sold to you would be false. You could even buy one of the traditional hooped caravans with window-sills decorated in lace borders and porcelain. The gypsies had no use for them any more; they lived in silver streamlined mobile homes now, with a tangle of aerials on the roof.

A lane ran between the fields and it had been closed off and turned into a race track for the horse and harness riders. They sprinted up and down the hill here, training for the races to be held towards the end of the fair. As I leant against the fence and watched, a RSPCA officer hurried over and said: 'is that horse giving birth?'

There was a mare lying down and licking her genitalia.

'No,' the RSPCA man said, 'it's just having a lick. I thought it might be giving birth.'

A horse and harness rushed past; a child was grabbed and whisked away. I asked the RSPCA man what had happened down at the river with the dead horse. 'There was a post mortem,' he said. 'The horse drowned all right. The bloke's been charged with excessive cruelty.'

I didn't envy this man his job here. His brief was to poke his nose in. He said, 'All I can do is try to make sure they don't use the whip too much. And then I can only ask them to stop. If we try to prosecute, the family gather round in a flash. And the police don't want to know; not unless it's something messy like that dead one in the river.'

But most of the animals were well looked after, he said. 'They look after them better than they look after themselves.' He patted Boogie. 'Hello boy,' he said. Boogie eyed him warily. He's suspicious of anyone in uniform, ever since the police picked him up for loitering and endorsed his dog licence.

I bought some fudge from a stall next to Gypsy Rose Lee's caravan. 'Palms read, fortunes told,' said the sign and advertised a list of celebrity clients such as Frank Ifield and Kevin Keegan. Inside sat a tubby and toothless old lady with a shy smile. The fact that she had two caravans made me wonder — did she tell two fortunes at once, flitting between the two, or had she sold the franchise? Then she clicked her tongue at Boogie and he was hauling me up the steps into the caravan.

'Shall I leave the dog outside?' I asked, but she was already peering into a ball, smoothing the surface. Her shawl fell over her eyes and she brushed it away with her brown wrinkled fingers.

'Just sit down,' she said. 'You have children, no?'

'Yes,' I answered, and suddenly wished I hadn't come up these steps. This was suddenly more than a joke. I had the feeling I had just passed over control of my life to this woman.

'Two children. Boys. Five and two,' I added. I didn't want any surprises on that front.

'You are away from them?' she said.

'Yes. I'm walking the Pennine Way actually, ha.' I was sweating. I was giving her information she didn't want. She brushed away clouds that hid her view.

'I see clouds,' she said.

'Been very good weather since I left. Hardly had any rain; haven't had to put my waterproofs on. . . .'

'I see clouds,' she repeated.

Of course, these were the clouds of the future that would rain fire and brimstone on me. This was the flood that was about to bowl me over, retribution for the smug face I'd had since Edale, for thinking the Pennine Way was a doddle. At this moment a mother of a ridge of low pressure was mustering mid-Atlantic, climbing into a meteorological catapult to be flung eastward, and it had my name on it.

'The clouds distort the way ahead. Cross my palm with silver.'

I gave her a pound coin. She said, 'It is very muddy and foggy. It is hard to see through. You are lost. You are looking round and thinking: which way do I go from here? You are worrying but there is no need to worry.'

'I'm not worrying.'

'You have everything you need. You must learn to be happy with it.'

'I am happy.'

'I don't think you are.'

'Yes I am.'

'That's not what it says here.'

Miss Lee sat back and looked out of the window. There was a silence. I wasn't sure if the session was over or not. Boogie whined. I said, 'Do you do dogs?'

'I beg your pardon?' said Miss Lee.

'Do you read their palms? I mean paws?'

Miss Lee thought about this momentarily. 'Yes,' she said. 'Of course I do dogs.'

I sat Boogie by her and she picked up his left paw. 'You are walking the Pennine Way,' she said.

Boogie stuck his tongue out.

'You don't like walking the Pennine Way,' she said.

''Course he does.'

'You would rather be home watching the telly.'

I said, 'I think you'll find he's going through a mid-life crisis.'

'There is only one mid-life crisis in this room and it is yours, mister.'

She turned Boogie's paw over. 'You will live to an old age. You have a big heart. You are a jolly chap. Good company, but you have to put up with a lot.'

'Him?'

'Do not worry.'

'He's not worried. What's he got to worry about?'

'Things will get better. I see a happy ending for you as well. That's £5.50 please.'

I paid up and she smiled without looking at me, then patted Boogie and blew her nose on a very pretty hanky.

We took the train back to Ribblehead and I found another bunkhouse to sleep in, right next to the Station Hotel. I went to the bar and had cottage pie with more mushy carrots.

In a corner a businessman and his secretary were sitting having a drink, whispering in each other's ear. He wore a suit, had baggy eyes and looked worried. She had a deep tan and wore pink shoes, and she held his hand and kept patting it. I heard her say, 'I don't need a bigger office.'

When he came to the bar for refills, he saw Boogie lying flat out. 'What have you been doing to him?' he asked.

When I told him we were walking the Pennine Way, he was amazed. 'What, you just set off with your dog, on your own?'

'Yes.'

'I'd love to do that. I'd love to leave everything behind. Just walk out of the door.'

'I am going back home afterwards,' I said.

'Just pick a path and follow it. No pressure. All you've got to think about is your next meal.'

'I do have some responsibilities.'

'You don't know how lucky you are. I'd love to do that more than anything in the world.'

'Why don't you?'

He shook his head and said, 'Don't ask,' then carried two vodkas back to the table.

A crowd from Leeds University came in, looking impossibly young. They took the place over. The pool table pockets clattered as they strode round posturing with their cues like rock singers, miming to the music from the juke box.

In a crowd like this there was nothing to do but sit in a corner. I caught myself missing Doug and Tony from Liverpool. I would have quite liked a good equipment discussion. But I would be almost a day behind them now.

I went to bed early, snuggled into my sleeping bag. I had the whole bunkhouse to myself and it was chilly. I lay there listening to a dripping tap. 'What would you do if you won the lottery Boogie, eh?' I said to him, and I pictured a limo pulling up outside and a chauffeur opening the door for Boogie, saying, 'You wanted the Kennomeat factory I understand, sir.'

I kept being woken by some kids running past my window and knocking at the door. Boogie barked but didn't impress anyone and in the end I got up to chase them away. But when I opened the door I found no-one.

I stood there gazing at the viaduct, its grey curves aglow now in the cold silver light of the full moon.

A sheep bleated; the wind picked up the dust in the pub car park. You didn't have to try very hard to hear a ghost train a-coming down that line.

I turned back to the bunkhouse, and then I saw a stick lying on the ground. I picked it up, threw it to the other side of the car park and said to Boogie,

'Fetch boy. Come on. Fetch. You can do it. I saw you do it.'

Boogie looked over his shoulder as if I must be talking to another dog.

'Come on. Off you go. Fetch. Fetch the bloody stick, will you! There's a good . . . oh, forget it.'

I returned to the Pennine Way again the next morning, although it didn't seem important to be following it any more. There were a number of Ways around these parts: the Dales Way, the Ribble Way, and they were all Pennine ways in their own way. I could have followed any one of them and been taken through lovely high Pennine country. To some walkers I'd met, the very idea of coming off the path was anathema; it would mean their attempt was flawed. But I was beginning to think that the Pennine Way could be whatever you wanted it to be as long as it headed north and went over hills. This morning it was just a path that led up and over to Hawes.

We climbed out of the Ribble valley, the day clear and crisp. Huge amounts of sky and hill dominated the view in every direction. Villages like Ribblehead and Horton had tried to make an impression on this bare landscape, but they had only achieved it on the map; they were just names. In the light of day they appeared lost and exposed against the wide backdrop of the Three Peaks. Their little houses huddled together for protection, looking as vulnerable as a Yorkshire version of Pompeii. Even the train looked uneasy today as it rattled through. The sound carried right across the valley, but it was a pathetic sound.

The path followed an old Roman military road, called the Cam High Road, along another lovely grassy track, like walking on a carpet. As usual I was aware of a huge history underfoot here, and now, with all these different Ways around, it struck me what a living history it was.

These paths had served their time as packhorse trails and military roads as and when they were needed, and now they had a role as recreational routes. They were part of the fight against stress and heart disease in the home and workplace, which made them just as viable and just as big a part of social history, as far as I could see.

Dodd Fell reared up ahead and we finally climbed to the top of a ridge that offered a fine panorama. To the north was Wensleydale and beyond rose Great Shunner Fell, while behind me were still those Three Peaks that had filled the vision for days now. I stood there in the wind, thinking how lucky I'd been with visibility, how I'd yet to miss out on one view, wondering how long this could go on for.

Ahead, a lad sat on the grass, with his trouser leg rolled up, flexing his knee. Boogie as usual performed the introductions with a, 'would you mind getting up because I particularly want to sniff that patch of ground you're sitting on?'

The lad moved over and Boogie decided he wasn't bothered.

This walker was tall and lean and he was walking the Pennine Way at high speed. He'd started in Edale four days after me and would finish about two weeks before me at the rate we were each going. He expected to complete the whole thing in ten days.

But now he was sitting on the grass nursing a twisted knee sustained coming down Penyghent. 'I was going too fast,' he said.

He was surprised to meet someone else walking the Pennine Way. 'I've met very few people,' he said. That was probably because he was past them in a flash.

He rolled his trouser leg down and said he'd walk with me into Hawes, but I quickly realised I'd never be able to keep up with him. He talked fast as well, talked about the variety of long distance paths in Britain. He was ticking them off, one a year: The West Highland Way, Offa's Dyke, The Cambrian Way. 'My book shelf is filling up with guides,' he said.

I took a look around me and saw we were coming down through Langstrathdale and a fine sweep of country, and I was missing it all. I didn't want to go this fast. I said to him, 'listen, I'm going to stop and . . . and . . . write some postcards.'

'Nice talking to you,' he said. 'It kept my mind off my knee.' And he was gone, out of sight with a single bound.

I sat looking into the sweep of Wensleydale, and wrote to my two boys in big letters so the eldest could read it: 'I have walked a hundred miles and eaten twelve fried eggs. One day you will walk the Pennine Way and have lots of fried eggs too.'

The village of Gayle is reached just before Hawes, and it's such a surprise when you're expecting a busy market town that it's an undiscovered delight. I leaned on the bridge over the Duerly Beck, a crystal clear piece of water which cascades through the village from on high. A teacher led his class of twelve-year-olds down the steps to the river bank and they sat there in a burst of sunshine, drawing wild flowers.

One lad said to me, 'I've got a dog like that.'

'Have you? What's his name?'

'Rambo.'

'That's a nice name.'

'He bit the head off next-door's chicken.'

'Did he?'

'The thing was running around with no head. Blood everywhere.'

It was market day in Hawes, the self-styled capital of

the Yorkshire Dales. I wanted to buy some Wensleydale cheese but I couldn't find any in the whole market. There was a factory somewhere in the town but not a lump of the stuff was for sale. Maybe you had to get here early. Seven o'clock in the morning it probably arrived on a wagon, there was a huge cheese rush and that was it for the day.

Instead there were lots of shoes and acrylic pullovers for sale; unlikely socks and unattractive underwear; a few jars of homemade jam and mint sauce. Hawes market had gone the way of most country town markets nationwide. There was a good turnout of tourists but there didn't seem much for them to do except read the menus in the café windows. Everyone breathed in as a huge coach bearing the words Majestic, The Great British Tour, squeezed between the buildings up the high street. The passengers looked down on Hawes from inside their fishbowl with blank faces. The coach slowed to a crawl as it hit cobblestones. The driver mouthed a curse at a motorist who clipped his wing mirror, then he hit tarmac again, put his foot down and The Great British Tour moved on.

I bought some lunch and tried to find a bench to sit down on in some area away from the road, but these all came with signs that said: 'Sorry, no dogs.' So we ended up outside the Tourist Information Office surrounded by cars.

There was a ropemaker's nearby where you could go and watch the ropemaker at work. A couple were debating whether to venture in or not:

'I don't know if it's worth it,' he said.

'It's free, Norman,' she replied.

'I know but. . . .'

'But what. . . ?'

'Well, he's only making rope.'

'I want to watch.'

'You know what these people are like.'

He knew that in the tourist business you rarely got

something for nothing. But he let her have her way; they were on holiday after all. 'I'm not buying any rope or nothing, mind,' he muttered as he followed her in.

I asked in the tourist office if there was anywhere to stay between Hawes and Keld and before I knew it, the woman at the desk had phoned up a guest house in the village of Thwaite and negotiated a price for bed and breakfast with evening meal. I never liked to book accommodation in advance in case I changed plans, but there didn't seem anywhere else to stay between here and Keld, and she had got me a good deal, so I said yes.

'You'll pass the highest waterfall in England at Hardrow,' she said with a smile rich in local pride. 'The dog will enjoy that.'

She was using the tourist officer's poetic licence here of course. Dogs are capable of many things, but an appreciation of scenery is, as far as I can tell, beyond them. It's certainly beyond Boogie. Offer him a meadow to play in or a car park and he'll take the car park every time. As it turned out he did enjoy Hardrow Force but this was because the way to the waterfall is through a pub, and if there's one place Boogie prefers to play in rather than a car park, it's a pub.

I'd imagined that the waterfall would have been off the beaten track, maybe even a spectacle that only walkers on the Pennine Way could reach. I certainly never expected to gain access to it through the public bar of the Green Dragon Inn in Hardrow, having coughed up 60 pence.

But there it was, across a neat lawn, cascading very gracefully over a limestone cliff. At ninety-six feet high it's no Niagara, but as far as beer garden attractions go it takes some beating.

Great Shunner Fell was the afternoon's exercise, a muscular hillside that blocked the way north. And yet the ascent was nowhere near as arduous as it looked. I

climbed slowly, feeling the sun on my face. The gradient
was steady and the views stretched back magnificently,
each step up producing another distant peak behind us
to the south. There was the path I'd followed that
morning, The West Cam Road. And then Penyghent
and Whernside reappeared like friends you've met on
holiday and already said goodbye to at the airport knowing
you're never going to see them again, and then you bump
into them five minutes later on the train and don't know
what to say.

I reached the top and found a German couple sitting on
a wall. They'd climbed this hill every day for the last three
days, they said, and each time the visibility had improved.
'Look,' she said, and pointed with her walking stick, 'They
are the Lake District far away to the west.'

She was probably right, but it was hard to concentrate
on any view with her husband standing next to you. He
was wearing a pair of striped boxer shorts pulled up high
over a belly which looked as though he'd swallowed a
beach ball for lunch. For reasons best known to himself he
wore his vest outside his shirt, and on his feet he sported
red baseball boots. His hat was covered with badges. He
stepped forward, stood to attention and pulled a packet of
sweets from his pocket, saying, 'Have a humbug.'

I'd walked over twenty miles already that day – the furthest
distance I'd covered. I was already tired, and now the
descent from Great Shunner was a killer, along a very
rough track, picking a route through broken boulders. I
was glad I was booked into a place, and in a guest house as
well. It was good to treat yourself now and again on these
treks. Splash out a bit. I walked with the image of the house
I'd be staying at growing ever more idyllic in my mind. It
would be stone with roses growing round the front door
and a stream running through the garden. A bright yellow

and blue room with a low window looking over meadows to the fells. A motherly host who didn't mind dog hairs and would insist I had second helpings of everything, and who didn't overcook her carrots.

Then there was Thwaite, far below and looking irresistible in the early evening sunlight. A yellow splash of wild flowers coloured the meadows, and every field had its own stone barn and was wrapped tightly within a stone wall.

On one of these walls I saw the lad I'd met earlier in the day, the Pennine Way speedster.

'How's the knee?' I asked.

'Not too good.'

'Are you stopping?'

'I'll wait a bit before I put up my tent by some stream.'

I was heading for a night of luxury but now I felt envious of him with his tent and everything he needed to survive on his back. I didn't want him to know that I was booked into a guest house with dinner pre-booked.

'How about you?' he asked.

'Oh, I'll bunk down in Thwaite probably.'

'I'll walk down with you. See if I can find a farmer.'

We walked down into the village. He wanted to find a farmer to ask permission to camp. He had done this every night since Edale, but I knew he would have loved just one night inside. It was stupid: a man with a tent who wanted to stay in a B&B, and a man who was booked to stay in a B&B wanting to sleep in a tent.

The village of Thwaite was as pretty as could be, with a post box, a bridge over a stripling river, a parish notice board and a farmhouse. And next to the farmhouse was the guest house I was booked in.

I looked at it and couldn't believe what I saw. At one time no doubt it had been a building like all others in the village, unpretentious and gentle on the eye. Now it had an extension and a big car park stuck on the back and an AA listed sign on the front. It was the last sort of place I wanted to stay at and I hesitated, wondering whether I could walk past and disown it. I certainly didn't want to let this camper know I was staying there.

But if you book somewhere and don't turn up, before you know it the Mountain Rescue are out looking for you, and then as I peered into the place a man in a black tie and a white shirt appeared and saw Boogie and said: 'Ah Mr Wallington. You're here just in time. Evening meal at six thirty. You've fifteen minutes.'

I couldn't look my friend the camper in the face. I put my head down and hurried into the guest house. A sign on the door said, No Dogs, maybe I could escape yet. 'Oh, don't worry about that,' my host said, as he handed me a key and pointed me up the stairs into the new wing.

Inside the room were tea making facilities and a built-in wardrobe. Boogie loved the place; he was padding round, all excitement, 'I knew this trip could be like this,' written over his face. If they'd had a vacancy for hotel dog he would have applied.

I lay on the bed and tried to enjoy it as well, but I couldn't. I was reminded of a motel in a motorway service station.

At 6.30 I was sitting in the dining room at a little table all to myself as the room filled. There were a number of Americans and Germans among the other guests, although I could tell the couple who sat near to me with their elbows on the table were English. They wore polyester clothes and spoke in whispers. Not that there was any need to say anything at all. The Americans were capable of doing all the talking.

'You look nice tonight,' said a man called Carl to the woman sitting opposite, 'now you've got the blood off.'

'It made a mess, didn't it?' she replied. 'I didn't expect it to spurt like that.'

I tried to work out what they were talking about. It sounded like some attraction they'd visited. But where could it be that tourists visited and got blood spurting over them? A café where you killed your own lunch. Not in the Dales surely?

'Your knife wasn't sharp enough if you ask me,' said the woman next to Carl.

'It was good fun though,' said Carl.

They were in a party of about ten and they talked in glowing terms of James Herriot – for this was the heart of James Herriot Country. That must have been it. They were on a James Herriot tour and it included a visit to a veterinary surgery where for five pound extra you were allowed to operate on an animal of your choice.

'Didn't James Herriot die?' said the woman who had had blood on her dress.

'No,' said the woman next to her. 'He couldn't have . . . I mean I'd have known.'

'I'm sure he died.'

The meal was a roast dinner with mushy carrots. Maybe mushy carrots were a Yorkshire delicacy. Maybe there had been a time when carrots were considered poisonous unless they were cooked to a pulp and the recipe had stuck. Or maybe it was me. I was a weirdo who liked his carrots with a bite. From now on I'd ask for my carrots rare. See if that made any difference.

I'd lost my appetite. I wrapped bits of meat and potato up for Boogie.

'Is the pork local?' asked a German at table six.

'Er . . . not exactly,' said the waitress.

'Good,' said the German.

The English couple were overwhelmed into silence. They had the mannerisms of puppets as they passed each other the condiments, and chewed every mouthful at great length before they swallowed. You expected their heads to crash into their plates at any moment.

The Americans talked continually of the places they had been on previous vacations. They seemed to belong to some sort of holiday club.

'Did you go on the trip to Belize last year?'

'No, we went to Honduras to look at ruins.'

Then from one table another English woman tried to join in. She leant across and said, 'Now be honest, what don't you like about England? Don't be embarrassed.'

The Americans smiled and one said, 'Oh we'd have to think about that,' and the English woman replied, 'Do you know, in York Minster they have a stained glass window as big as a tennis court?'

'Yeah, I knew that,' said Carl.

I wondered if I was the only person walking the Pennine Way ever to have stayed here. The Pennine Way can be anything you want it to be I'd been telling myself, but closeted in this dining room it was hard to think that the path went past the front door.

'Do you want ice cream with your Queen's pudding?' asked the waitress.

I felt as though I was trapped in the corner of a stage, in some hideous drama, and I didn't know my lines. I remember feeling less lonely on the top of Black Hill. The Americans felt sorry for me because I was on my own, that was clear. They didn't want me to feel left out. They kept smiling at me and making comments like: 'aren't the flowers in the meadows pretty?'

Then in the middle of eating his Queen's pudding and ice cream, Carl turned his chair round and beamed at me: 'didn't I see you come in with a dog?'

'Yes,'

'Well, where the hell is it?'

'Watching Channel 4 news.'

He laughed, thinking I was joking. I asked him if they were just travelling round or what? and was surprised when he said they were all walking the Coast to Coast path. It cut across the Yorkshire Dales and the Pennine Way not far from here. Carl said: 'We heard about this little guest house and wanted to stay here, so we all rented a bus.'

'We're all from LA,' said the woman next to him. 'But we tackled those bogs, no mistake.'

When I said I was walking the Pennine Way, they nodded knowledgeably. 'We researched that one,' said Carl. 'It was the preference of a number of our group. But there was a young girl murdered on that path last year.'

That shut everyone up. Even the Germans on table six.

'So where to tomorrow?' I asked, breaking the silence.

'Oh tomorrow is a layover day. We've got the bus and we're going to go into Muker and visit the facilities.'

Dinner seemed to have taken for ever. Maybe that was why they served it so early because there was only one waitress and she took hours to get round the dining room. Finally she announced: 'coffee will be served in the lounge,' and I could stand it no longer. I set off to visit the facilities in Muker myself for a beer.

The footpath went through the glorious meadows I had seen from Great Shunner, and this cheered me up, but then I saw a tent engulfed by flowers nestled up against a dry stone wall, and there was the walker with the bad knee washing himself in the river below. I felt annoyed with myself all over again for staying in the stupid guest house, and I hurried past him embarrassed to be seen, thinking: I'm going to get myself a tent. I am.

5. *Duck à l'orange* in Teesdale

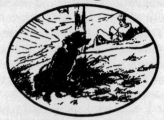

The news feature on Radio Cleveland the next morning was a worrying one. The highest suicide rate in the country was to be found among north country sheep farmers, notably those in the Yorkshire Dales.

The reasons for this hadn't been established, although financial problems were most likely to blame. Sheep farming could be a precarious business, the wolf daily at the door in the threat of bankruptcy.

These were proud folk, many from generations of shepherds working the same land. Now they were dependent on government subsidy, and were being undermined by red tape from Brussels, to the extent that for some suicide was ultimately preferable to the humiliation of going bust. The older farmers were said to be especially at risk.

Loneliness was also a factor. Technology had reduced the need for farm labour, and farmers often worked on their own twelve hours a day. The Royal Mail van was sometimes the only visitor.

Another theory was that continued use of sheep dip caused severe depression and 'suicidal thoughts'.

The very idea that it was common for farmers to suffer severe depression made me feel depressed. You looked at the glorious country around Thwaite and Muker and you couldn't imagine anywhere more efficacious. As I'd walked down Great Shunner Fell the previous evening the view had been uplifting, like walking into a land of milk and honey. I wrote something soft in my notebook about how the display of spring and summer really looks like a miracle in these dales, Wensleydale and Swaledale.

And yet to those who had to work and live here, to the very people who kept this land so beautiful, apparently it was a short hop to suicide. The face of a Swaledale sheep was the National Park logo, but behind it now I could see the shadow of a farmer with a shotgun in his mouth.

It was the kind of news I didn't want to share with people. I couldn't bring myself, for example, to tell the young woman I met outside Thwaite who was skipping through the meadows on Kisdon Hill with a smile on her face and her arms outstretched. 'What a day to be alive on!' her body language said, to which the reply: 'yes, and did you know 500 farmers committed suicide last year?' would have sounded morose.

Her smile was for me, her outstretched arms were for Boogie. He leapt up and slapped a kiss on her nose and would have rolled about in the grass with her if I hadn't pulled him off.

'I love animals,' she said.

'That's lucky.'

'What sort is he?'

'He's a dog. . . .'

She was American and another James Herriot fan. In fact she was walking the Herriot Way, a five day hike around the Dales. I remarked on the number of Americans I was meeting here and she said: 'James Herriot is very popular in the United States. After his TV show was on lots of people wanted to become vets. I wanted to become a vet.'

She tickled Boogie and he rolled over and spread his legs: bit lower, up a bit, down, oh that's it, oh that's lovely.

'The problem is I'm allergic to dogs,' she sighed.

'Oh dear.'

'They make me nauseous if I spend too long with them.'

She asked where I was walking to and when I told her she pulled a face and said, 'A lone woman hiker was murdered on the Pennine Way a year or so ago.'

I hadn't wanted to spread that story either. I didn't even know if it was true, although it seemed to be common knowledge among Americans.

'I didn't want to do the Pennine Way because of that,' she said. 'It's a pity, one person goes and spoils it for everyone else.'

I walked on with murder on my mind, although it seemed doubtful to me that the murderer would confine himself to the Pennine Way. If he did have it in for ramblers he could chose from a variety of paths round here.

The Long Distance Footpath Murders. It was a good, shocking headline. You don't associate rambling with homicide, or crime of any sort for that matter. And yet muggers could do good business in the summer months on the Pennine Way. Most walkers going the whole distance would carry a hundred pound in cash and during the season there were probably ten a day, and so for members of the criminal fraternity who could use a map and compass here was a regular holiday job.

But what was I thinking about? It wouldn't be money the muggers would be after. They'd leap out from behind their gritstone yelling: 'your Gore-tex jacket, or your life.'

Some murderer had been at work on the path that morning: a fox perhaps, or some bird of prey with a taste for rabbits. Whatever it was it modelled itself on Jack the Ripper. Disembowelled corpses lay at regular intervals on the path, their intestines smeared over the grass like some omen. Boogie stepped round them with disgust. If he had to live off his wits he'd have problems. He could maybe hold up a grocery store and steal a tin of dog food, but then he'd have to kidnap someone to help him open it.

The path followed the contour of the dale towards the village of Keld, past the ubiquitous barns, and always with fine views down onto the River Swale as it flowed with a throaty enthusiasm from its head. It was another billowing morning, clouds spinning across the sky like escaped bedding, a perfect walking day and I was the only person on the hill.

I came down to the river before we reached Keld just to have a look at the waterfall that was signposted. In the end though I spent the rest of the morning there, messing about in a series of falls much more impressive than the more famous one back at Hardrow, and all hidden from the path by the cliffs. I felt very lucky to be a walker in this place. No one else could reach here. It was the loveliest, most secret spot of the whole walk and I wanted to stop a while and do something with the falls as a backdrop, have a picnic or maybe even a swim. There was a clear, cool pool at the bottom of one fall that said: 'go on, get naked and jump in me!' So I took my socks off and stuck my feet in the water and it was so cold it was like an electric shock. Instead I decided to do my laundry, pummelling my socks with a rock, the way Mexican peasants do in movies.

We scrambled upstream over stepping stones to Catrake Force, Boogie's nose quivering in the waves of wild garlic we waded through. The whole gorge began to smell like a bistro.

We played around in the water for a while, a game called Boogie-sticks, a pointless exercise where I throw sticks for him and he ignores them completely. Finally we emerged in Keld with wet feet and big appetites.

'Are you Pennine Waying it?' said a voice behind me. I turned round to see a lad sitting on the bench next to a big rucksack.

Pennine Waying it? 'Yes,' I replied. 'I am Pennine Waying it. How about you? Are you Pennine Waying it?'

'Oh I'm Pennine Waying it all right,' he said with verve. He was also Offa's Dyking it. In fact he was Aberdeen to Gloucestering it on foot for charity. The Pennine Way was merely his middle stretch. Aberdeen was where he studied; Gloucester was where he lived. He was walking home. Simple.

Twenty days he'd been on the road, and twenty more to go. We did lunch and talked of underwear on the footpath, the colour of crisp bags, the special needs sailing club he was ràising money for. And I thought I was actually going to have an encounter with a hiker that didn't involve a discussion on equipment, but then he spotted my socks hanging on my belt to dry and he said, 'interesting.'

'What is?'

'Woollen, rag stitch socks. That's very interesting.'

Interesting isn't the word I would use to describe my socks, or anyone's socks for that matter. I gazed quizzically at him for an explanation and he opened his rucksack and pulled out a pair of his own socks. Nothing interesting about them either, I thought, but I was wrong.

'Synthetic, loopstitch,' he said, offering me a closer look.

'Really.'

'Ragstitch is generally better because it keeps its pile all day. Loopstitch tends to flatten out after a few hours of walking.'

Was he saying he was impressed by my socks?

'However yours are woollen and wool makes your feet sweat. You need synthetic to keep the moisture away from your foot.'

Now he was insulting my socks.

'It's just that you don't often see woollen ragstitch.'

'No,' I said, nodding in agreement. I was happy with my socks, but I wasn't going to stand up and defend them in an argument with someone who really knew his socks.

The Coast to Coast path crossed the Pennine Way at Keld. The former seemed to have overtaken the latter as the fashionable hike to do and I imagined here would be a walkers' crossroads, with cafés and accommodation, bulletin boards where hikers could leave messages, a second-hand hiking shop, a pub called the Wainwright Arms. But the lad from Aberdeen and I had it to ourselves. And it was delightful, another one of those villages I wrote down on the back page of my notebook in the places-to-come-back-to column.

I said to him, 'Have you had much rain?'

'Loads. Pissed down in the Cheviots.'

'I haven't had any yet,' I said.

And he laughed as if I was joking. So I laughed as if I was joking too. But then I said, 'No, I mean it.'

He looked at me sternly. 'What, no rain the whole way?'

'No.'

'From Edale to here?'

'Yes.'

'Oh, I wouldn't like that.'

Boogie and I climbed out of the treelined cradle of Swaledale and quickly the gargling of its river was gone and we were crossing Stonesdale Moor. With a familiar ease that was always quite frightening the Pennine Way slipped from gentle beauty back into an all-consuming bleakness. The comfort of the barns and wildflowers was gone. The sky became the colour of ice, and I felt lost and remote once more. It seemed unthinkable that an hour earlier I'd been contemplating a swim.

It always amazed me to bump into people just when

I was feeling so isolated, but there over a rise came
a man wearing a balaclava and gloves and pushing a
mountain bike.

He was cycling coast to coast. 'Went up to my handlebars
in a peat bog yesterday,' he said with glee.

In fact he wasn't cycling coast to coast so much as
carrying his bike coast to coast, but he seemed happy
enough. He had the exuberance of all these walkers and
campers and cyclists. I couldn't remember meeting one
who was dejected enough to want to go home, or was
willing to say what an awful time he was having. Everyone
on the path had a mental resilience that bordered on the
psychotic.

At times that was exactly what you needed, as when
I climbed to the top of Tan Hill and was confronted by
what could only be a mirage. I was surrounded by raw and
rolling moor and yet rising out of the desolation ahead was
a single building – and it was a pub.

Ignore it and it will go away, I told myself, and I
scratched my eyes and expected it to disappear. But then
I could see smoke coming from its chimney, and the path
turned into a track that led unerringly to its front door. It
really was a pub. It was The Tan Hill Inn, the highest,
loneliest pub in England.

This was once a packhorseman's crossroads. It was also
a lead miner's haunt, and the front of the inn still retains
the look of a rough shelter. But times have changed. Gone
are the days when you couldn't get served here without
a filthy face and an industrial disease. If you ask for tea
and biscuits now instead of a beer no-one laughs at you
or calls you a cissy. And if you walk through to the rear
of the building you'll even find a function room, rather
gracelessly tacked onto the original building but advertised
as the place to have the wedding of your dreams.

You can imagine couples flying away to the Caribbean

to get married. Balmy nights on tropical beaches and snaps of the bride and groom under a coconut palm have a certain glamorous gloss. But to come to the top of Tan Hill to tie the knot requires an altogether different interpretation of romance, a much muddier sort.

The staff don't see this as a problem of course. A stone-flagged floor, two coal fires (always lit, as a notice proudly boasts), and a selection of Theakston's hand-pulled beers is the epitome of *l'amour* in these parts. When I showed an interest, I was seen by a smart young woman who tried to impress upon me the ease of it all. How the pub would arrange for the registrar to come up from Richmond; how they could offer a selection of buffets to fit all pockets: 'chicken drumsticks, petit crolines in three flavours, and vol au vents,' she beamed. 'There's also unlimited parking.'

The first couple were due to arrive the following weekend. 'They met in this bar right here,' the woman said. She was hoping the idea would catch on with Pennine Way walkers. 'You can get married here, then have your honeymoon walking the Pennine Way,' she suggested.

'And get divorced in Kirk Yetholm' I added, but that didn't go down very well.

Boogie was busy auditioning for the position of traditional pub dog lying in front of the fire asleep. But his time was up and anyway he wasn't a match for the other four-legged slobs gathered round the hearth in comatose positions. They were old luvvies who lay there scorching themselves and only barked when another bucket of coal was needed. A yawn, a scratch and an erotic dream, and that was their exercise for the day.

I dragged Boogie outside. Ahead of us was a grim piece of moorland that needed to be navigated while we still had the energy. This was Sleightholme Moor and it spread amorphously away from Tan Hill into a featureless distance. No-one would hear you scream out there.

We followed a moorland river, the Frumming Beck. Cloud still raced across the sky, although in the distance to the east it was clear blue and the way that the hills gave way to much lower ground really gave the impression we were walking towards the coast. I could hear waves, for heaven's sake; I could taste an ice cream wafer. Another mirage perhaps. Everyone had said navigation over Sleightholme was tricky, and if you strayed off the path you'd be at the bottom of one of the many abandoned mine shafts before you could say, *arrrgh*! I stopped and studied the map and tried to take a compass bearing, but there was little to take a bearing off. One section on the map was simply and depressingly called The Bog.

The Tan Hill Inn was quickly a dot in the rear view mirror. The thought of being in their function room nibbling prawn crolines, wearing a carnation in my jacket and saying I do, was suddenly very comforting. Then it was gone and I was on my own again, and ahead of me was a pair of jeans lying in a puddle of peat. It was as if someone had got stuck in the mire and been pulled out minus their pants. These discarded pieces of clothing were becoming puzzling. From underwear they had now progressed to leisure wear. Maybe they all belonged to the same person. Maybe two walkers were doing the Pennine Way tearing each other's clothes off.

I walked with my head down for an hour or more until in the distance I could see a farm, then a farmer out in his field putting up a new gate. I reached out to the first human I'd seen since lunchtime.

'Blowy isn't it,' I said, and wondered if I'd contracted that syndrome common to walkers that makes them state the obvious whenever they meet strangers.

The farmer grunted and looked away. Misery, I thought,

and marched on. But then it occurred to me he was probably
clinically depressed, and the worst thing I could have done
was try to cheer him up with small talk about the weather.
He was probably striding back to his farm right now and
attaching a hosepipe to an exhaust. I wondered whether I
should turn back and offer to counsel him, get him to sit
down and make a list of all the good things in his life on
one side of the paper and all the bad things on the other.

A busy road was visible far into the distance, sunlight
glinting off metal roofs. We were heading into Bowes, a
town with a castle, a Roman history, literary connections,
and a bypass. The perfect place to stay the night. But it took
me hours to get there. I kept losing the path and ending up
walking through farmyards trying to find an exit. We'd turn
a corner and a mad sheepdog would come bounding out at
us. It would leap for Boogie's throat and then bounce back
as its chain reached full length.

Bowes just never seemed to get any nearer. I grew
frustrated, and then when I couldn't find the bridge to
cross the River Greta I lost my temper. If a hiker had
greeted me at that point with a jolly 'are you Pennine
Waying it?' I'd have told him to go and boil his head.

Instead a herd of cattle bore the brunt of my mood. As
we climbed over a stile into a field, about twenty of them
came hurtling across at Boogie and I couldn't be bothered
to run away so I yelled profanities at them. I was as surprised
as anyone when they stopped in their tracks, and from then
on whenever cows charged Boogie or me, I shocked them
with foul language and it did the trick.

When I did finally get to Bowes I was in one bad sulk.
The castle dated back to the twelfth century but looked to
me like some glum lump McAlpine had put up. The town
appealed to the Romans because of its strategic position in
the Stainmore Gap, but it was just a grey village threaded
along a straight road as far as I could see. The literary

connection was to do with Dickens, a building on the main street once housed a school which inspired Dotheboys Hall in *Nicholas Nickleby*. It was shut, though, and a gale was blowing down the main street – a street which had 'one horse' written all over it.

I sat on a bench and filled my face with a bar of chocolate and when a man came and patted Boogie and said, 'Bet he's good company,' I replied, 'Oh he's no end of fun! We play cards or chess or something every night. And at weekends he brings out his Travel Scrabble for dogs. Or sometimes we just stay up late and discuss Bosnia.'

'Mine's just the same,' said the man.

But if I wasn't enamoured with Bowes, Bowes wasn't exactly taken with me, offering nowhere to stay. I asked passers-by but they shook their heads and said try Barnard Castle, four miles away. When someone offered me a lift there I jumped at the offer.

The next four miles were the most dangerous of the whole walk as a young lad with a fierce moustache put his foot down and drove like a madman into Barnard Castle. A farmer with nothing to live for, I assumed, and he was going to take me with him.

In fact he was a soldier and he was on his way to Newcastle. I didn't want to chat to him in case he lost concentration, but he kept turning to me and telling me how he had to get back home before eight because he was seeing his girlfriend who got angry if he didn't pick her up on the dot, and she was a cracker and worth hanging on to, 'cos he'd been in Germany and he knew what life was like without a good woman, and what was I doing leaving my woman at home on her own, and what the hell was the attraction of walking the Pennine Way, and was it me or my dog who smelt so bad?

I just made comments like: 'Goodness me, this is a fast road isn't it?' and 'Is that speedometer right?' and 'I bet there are lots of accidents along here,' but he didn't take any notice. We came flying down the hill into Barnard Castle at such a speed my boot made a dent in the footwell. When I came to get out I couldn't find Boogie. He was under the back seat with his paw over his eyes, shaking.

The soldier drove away with a screech and left me with my heart thumping on the edge of a town I'd never heard of. I didn't even know what county I was in.

Barnard Castle. Well there was the castle, right in front of me in a commanding position beloved of castles looking over a river, The Tees. And there was a finely pointed bridge leading to a gateway through the old town walls. What a welcome! They'd let down the drawbridge for me.

I found a place to stay near the river. An old woman with a bad chest patted Boogie until his head ached and then showed me to the room and told me that showers were ten pence extra. 'There's no plug for the bath either,' she added. 'But we are very central.'

I wasn't bothered about washing. I wanted food. I gave Boogie his meal and left him watching Coronation Street with our landlady, and I hit the town. It was eight o'clock and everything was closed, and yet in Barnard Castle the closed shop windows are very appealing. There's little sign of chain-store syndrome here. There's even a beautiful petrol station – an oxymoron if ever there was one – right in the middle of town, the equivalent of a free house. No BP or Esso signs here, just a smartly painted racing green frontage, some wrought iron awnings, and a window display that is half motor accessories and half ladies' and gentlemen's leisurewear.

I ended up in the Golden Gate Chop Suey House Takeaway, sitting on the window sill in a big empty room, eating king prawns and watching a kingsize TV as motorbikes roared up the main street.

'What county are we in?' I asked the woman serving.

She wasn't sure about me. 'Durham,' she replied.

Durham, of course. I should have guessed by the north east accent. A short car ride and suddenly everyone was sounding different. I said, 'So. What happens in Barnard Castle?'

'Nothing.'

'Nothing eh? Good. What, nothing at all?'

'There's the pubs and that's about it. And there's the Bowes Museum.'

She wasn't doing the town justice. Having surfaced here from the emptiness of Sleightholme Moor, I felt at once comfortable with Barnard – quickly getting on first name terms with the town. I felt as if I'd tumbled off the back of something and landed back in civilisation. With its well-swept high street and a lovely river setting this was the most sophisticated place I'd passed through.

I went back to my lodgings and took Boogie out round the park. 10.30 and kids were still playing football on this midsummer's evening. I thought how the nicest times of this walk had all occurred by accident, when I'd jumped on something and been taken along. It was easy to feel self-contented here, lost in England somewhere.

An old man with a beagle walked up to me and sat down, leaning on his walking stick. He clicked his false teeth together and looked at the kids. 'They're still playing football look.'

I tried to think of a statement-of-the-obvious of equal brilliance, but couldn't.

He stroked his dog with hands corrugated with veins. 'Good old Charlie,' he said. 'I wouldn't walk anywhere if it wasn't for Charlie. He gets me out of the house.'

We sat in silence and watched the football. I admitted to myself that maybe I'd used Boogie as an excuse to come on this walk, to get me out of the house. I patted him and a cloud rose from his coat. It was him who smelt awful.

The old man sighed and muttered, 'Oh well,' as if he was about to go, but then he said, 'I'm glad you're here.'

'Why's that?'

''Cos you can help me up.'

He gave me his arm and I helped him to his feet. 'It's going to get warmer,' he said. 'I can feel it in my legs,' and he and Charlie wobbled slowly home.

Later I lay in bed feeling cosy and happy and heard church bells strike midnight, a comfort to any traveller in a strange town. Next thing I knew they were striking seven and I was coming down for breakfast.

I could hear a fried egg crackling in the kitchen and smell hot fat. My host appeared wearing an apron and dragging her slippers behind her. She plonked my breakfast on a mat of the Houses of Parliament, put the *Sun* down next to me and said, 'Linford Christie's mother's dead.'

Everyone in Barnard Castle spoke of the Bowes Museum and its wonderful collection, and how I shouldn't leave until I had paid a visit. The woman I stayed with said: 'It's wonderful. I should know, I used to work there. I'll watch your dog.'

So I left Boogie with her on the couch reading the *Sun*, and walked to the huge French chateau on the edge of town, built a hundred years ago specifically to house the art collection of John Bowes and his French actress wife Josephine.

The concierge glanced at my boots and would have said something witty but he couldn't think of anything. So he made no comment at all and I climbed to the top of the house and worked my way down.

I was amazed to find El Greco's *The Tears of St Peter* here, as well as works by Goya in a large Spanish collection. There were Italian, French and Flemish art rooms, and huge amounts of furniture and porcelain displayed in period settings. I stood looking at Wooded Landscape With Figures by Jacob Van Esselenms (1626–1687) and realised that until now the nearest I'd come to an artistic experience on the Pennine Way had been a pint of Theakston's Old Peculier.

The silver swan is the centrepiece of the Bowes Museum, a lifesize musical, clockwork bird, that once wound up performs an elaborate mechanical routine. Or so the guide book said. Visitors crowded round at the appointed time. An attendant put his hat on and asked us to stand back while he wound the device up. Then he pressed the start button and stood clear.

The swan shivered and made a series of staccato movements for twenty seconds as it preened itself. Then it bent down and picked up a silver fish which took another twenty seconds and then it resumed its original position and stopped dead. The attendant moved the clock hands for the next performance on to 4 pm and the crowd dispersed and that was that. 'Swans don't eat fish. Do they?' whispered a man in shorts.

Shorts! I went outside. Shorts weather indeed, warm and sunny. I hurried back to my lodgings to pick up Boogie and we headed through town towards the river. I wasn't going to return to Bowes to pick up the Pennine Way, I'd decided. I had my eyes on another diversion. I'd discovered that a path followed the River Tees upstream and would take us back to the Pennine Way about ten miles to the north. I liked the idea of walking alongside water on this fine day. The forecast was good, just the weather for camping – which was fortunate, because as I walked down through the castle grounds and found the river path, my pack was six pounds heavier with a cheap and nasty tent.

You think of the River Tees as an industrial waterway,

rolling through dockyards to a wide, discoloured mouth before it dumps itself into the grey North Sea. You forget that like all rivers it sprung to earth as pure as any newborn.

Downstream from Barnard Castle it widens into murky waters and rolls through Darlington, Middlesbrough and Stockton, but upstream it's an adolescent river throwing itself over falls for fun. Boogie took one look at the rich peaty brown water and jumped straight in. Then he jumped straight out again with a 'Was that you who pushed me?'

The path along the north bank was narrow and shrouded by trees, and it rose and fell as the river passed through gorges and opened out into water meadows. This was a much more civilised sort of walk. I was wearing shorts and a hat for the sun, and passing through villages where men bent under the bonnets of their cars with the radio on, women cut the grass with hover mowers and old folk sat around greens on benches donated by the WI. In Cotherstone I asked a woman where the public phone was and she said, 'it used to be right there. . . .', and pointed to where it used to be but wasn't now.

'. . . . but yoofs got hold of it,' she explained. 'So they moved it up there.' And she pointed to where it was now but where you still couldn't see it.

'Where?' I asked.

"Bout a mile up there. Half a mile for you. Yorkshire miles mind, not Durham miles.'

By coming into Cotherstone I'd crossed back into Yorkshire.

'Are Yorkshire miles longer or shorter than Durham miles?' I asked.

'Longer.'

I found the phone and it was out of order. I only wanted to call home because I'd remembered where the dustbags for the vacuum cleaner might be. But maybe I shouldn't have bothered. My family could look after themselves; they could cope without me; they could live without dustbags.

The path along the river bank petered out and so I had to pick my way along using the map. But this was real rambling, I told myself. Picking your way cross-country, not just following a designated path. My map was criss-crossed with a network of green dotted rights-of-way that led anywhere and everywhere. This was walking as a means of transport. I began to feel smug, and that, I should have known from experience, is a dangerous way to feel.

One minute I was striding along a trail, the next I was standing in a tangle of brambles and barbed wire with no sign of anyone ever having walked this way before. I pressed on, using a stick as a machete, Boogie keeping so fast to my heels I kept kicking him in the chin. It was hopeless though; I was having to hack a passage. I came through the brambles to find myself in a field of barley or something, and now there was no sign of a footpath. I walked round the edge, but then I couldn't find a way out on the other side. I climbed over the fence in the end and spent the best part of an hour blazing a trail through a wilderness of nettles, trying to convince myself this was the way to Middleton-on-Tees.

Eventually I crawled under a hedge and found myself on a road which was busy and had no pavement, and seemed to be the route grocery van drivers used when their girlfriend had just left them and they wanted to take it out on innocent pedestrians.

I had to jump into a hawthorn to avoid a Leyland Daf, and I sat there thinking: bollocks to real rambling. Picking one's way cross-country with a map is a nice idea, but hopelessly flawed unless paths are well-used, and you don't have to link them together with roads, and you go through scenery that's good to look at. At least designated long distance paths like the Pennine Way are created with those criteria in mind.

We reached Middleton bridge and turned into the town. Like most communities in these parts, Middleton was an old lead mining centre that had thrived in the nineteenth century when it had a population many times larger than today. Now the town sat on its benches and waited for the next boom, looking in all directions, not knowing where it would come from. Tourism had poked its nose in and sniffed around, but as yet this part of the country looked beautifully unspoilt. Who came to County Durham for their holidays?

I was going to find somewhere to camp that night but I decided to wait until a little later, when I could be more inconspicuous. I sat in a pub and bought a packet of crisps that might or might not have contained a £10,000 winner's token. The barmaid was watching TV but she turned and saw me open the packet. 'If I win £10,000 will you let me take you away from all this?' I asked.

'You what?'

'Nothing.'

I didn't win and she went back to watching *Heartbeat*, the TV series about a policeman set in a Yorkshire moorland village. She was starstruck. How she would have loved a TV series to be filmed in this town, and then she could serve drinks to film stars, and she'd get to know them, and she'd have their autographed photos on the wall: 'to Debbie, thanks for everything, love Crispin,' and maybe get a walk-on role and be discovered and. . . .

The adverts came on. The dog from the complete dog food advert bounded across the screen like a gymnast, fresh from a session with his personal stylist. Boogie hid under the seat. I said to him, 'I think you'd be more of a complete dog if we brushed your hair differently. The dog in the advert has got a ridgeback parting, and a sort of "wash and go" cut. Your hair is more . . . the messy look.'

The barmaid glanced in the mirror behind the bar and smacked her lips at herself. I said, 'What's the weather forecast, any idea?'

'No, sorry,' she said, and switched on a smile.

'Not rained for while.'

'I heard that weather guru on the radio, from Thirsk.'

'Oh yes.'

'He says when it rains it's going to flood.'

Outside a number of beat-up cars pulled up and about twenty travellers tumbled out. 'Leftovers from Appleby,' said the barmaid and she pulled up her sleeves.

They filed into the lounge bar. They looked like one big family: five-year-olds to eighty-year-olds.

'How much is a pint of John Smith's?' asked one man with a carnation in his coat.

'One pound forty,' said the barmaid

'Never. You can get it for half that price down the road.'

'How much is the whisky?' said a man with a hole in his hat.

'One twenty-five a shot.'

'I can get it for a fiver a bottle, woman!'

They questioned everything, paid up reluctantly and sat down. But they were a restless bunch. The kids grabbed the pool cues and tried to get the pool balls out without paying. A girl came to the bar and said she'd put money in the juke box but it had swallowed it. When the barmaid got it to work the girl put on the old Cher song 'Gypsies Tramps and Thieves', and tried to get the older ones to dance. The pub was suddenly one big party.

'Oi darlin?' – The barmaid wanted to watch her programme but they'd come for a second round – 'I've collected all the glasses. I'm doing your job for you, look love. That's a pound off for sure.'

The barmaid sighed and switched off the TV.

I went back to The Tees and walked for a way upstream until I found a good place to camp in a small clearing, a short distance from the river. My tent was cheap and ugly and I was immediately suspicious of it because I was able to erect it in minutes. But it was a shelter, and by the look of the sky it was all I would need. There was no wind and it felt warm enough to sleep out under the stars.

Boogie watched me with disbelief as I took great pleasure in washing in the brown peaty stream. His look said: what's the idea? There were nice lodgings back there in that nice town. There were beds and fried breakfasts and living rooms with snaps of the family on the mantelpiece and magazine racks and TVs and plumped-up cushions. We could have stayed there for £14.50, showers extra. Why sleep in a tent? Are you mad?

'Dinner,' I announced and tore open my packet of *Duck à l'orange* performance food. I boiled some water and poured it over the contents and then sat waiting for it to rehydrate. The sky grew starry. The river cleared its throat. A man in the living room of a semi-detached on the outskirts of Darlington opened a packet of biscuits and Boogie pricked his ears. It was the kind of evening to savour.

I was camping in Durham, for goodness' sake. I'd always pictured Durham as the A1, coal mines and run down housing estates with permanently wet pavements – and yet here I was camping in the most unspoilt corner of England I'd ever visited, and the night was starry and warm.

I looked at dinner. Dinner looked back at me. I don't know what I'd been imagining but it didn't look like *Duck à l'orange* to me. It looked remarkably like Boogie's complete dog food.

'Complete instant lightweight meal for people on the move', I read the packet for reassurance. That was me and Boogie, on the move, no strings, footloose, going places, going to Kirk Yetholm. 'High protein', the packet went on: 'wholesome, nutritious, high energy'. So why was it smelling of boiled tennis balls?

I spooned some on the plate and tasted it, then tasted some more, then some more. This wasn't because it tasted good, it was because it tasted of nothing. And when I say it tasted of nothing I mean it had captured the taste of nothing wonderfully. This was how I had always imagined nothing would taste. And such a strong taste of nothing was it that no matter what you added, it managed to make that taste of nothing too. Wholemeal bread – nothing. Lump of cheese – nothing. Slice of banana – nothing. I kept tasting it until I realised I was full. . . . of nothing. Then I offered the remains to Boogie. He ate it all in one mouthful, and gave me his, 'wow! that was delicious, any more?' face, the one he gives you when you feed him anything from a mixed grill to a worming tablet.

I went and sat by the water and washed in the brown peaty stream. I pulled out *Wuthering Heights*. Halfway into the journey and I was up to page forty-six. I read page forty-seven and started to yawn.

Darkness fell and the moon appeared, then caught me looking at it and hurried behind a cloud again. Was that a cloud bank mustering to the west? Camping was asking for trouble after all. Camping was daring the elements. I checked my ropes and pegs and crawled into the tent.

Boogie and I spent five minutes kicking each other as we wrestled for space. I discovered it was his breath that was the root of his hygiene problems. Lying next to him was like sleeping with a walrus. After ten minutes I'd had enough. I hauled him out of bed and back down to the river, and shoved my tooth brush in his mouth.

'This is what it's all about kid. Getting back to basics. Peeling back the layers and finding the youthful spirit within. Man and dog cleaning their teeth together in the great outdoors. Just look at that tartar. When you get back home you should start flossing as well.'

Back in the tent I lay there singing 'Gypsy Tramps and Thieves': 'I was born in the wagon of a travelling show, mama used to dance for the money they'd throw. . . .' I fell asleep and dreamed wildly. I was on a mountain and looking over to another peak, the next one I would have to climb. But it was raining furiously and there was a rising flood in the valley. A party of ramblers appeared and I said hello to them all but then they walked down the hill and were washed away.

Boogie woke me with a strange bark and a kick. He was dreaming too, and when he dreams it is all action. He makes noises you've never heard a dog make before. His face contorts into grimaces and luxurious smiles. His little legs scamper and every so often his entire body jolts. His dream looked like a much better one than mine. His tail was thumping and his lip was quivering. He was dreaming that he hadn't been dragged out on the Pennine Way. He'd been left at kennels where there'd been a mix up and he'd been put in a cage with all the bitches on heat.

I picked up *Wuthering Heights* and was soon asleep again. This time I dreamed I was in a house, a strange house and I was wandering round opening doors and finding empty rooms. A door slammed and I woke again, and suddenly felt nervous. Had the door slammed in my dream or was the noise from outside. A clap of thunder? I unzipped the tent and peeped out. The moon and stars had gone, a wind was picking up. There was a queue of clouds to the west. I could definitely smell rain. It wouldn't be long now. I got out my waterproofs and stuck them under my pillow, almost relieved that the tension would soon be over. I picked up *Wuthering Heights* again.

Next time I woke, it was six hours later and the book was still propped up on my chest. Light was playing on the corners of the tent. The sound of insects could be heard above the river. I pulled back the flaps and saw a perfect summer's morning. I felt full of joy; then I felt cheated; then I felt depressed. What did I have to do to be taken seriously? I had pitted myself against the elements and the elements couldn't be bothered with me. What else could I do except post my waterproofs home? This lack of rain was becoming a big problem.

We had joined the Pennine Way again, or rather the Pennine Way had joined us as it came down from the hills to meet the path along The Tees.

The trail along the bank was a stroll, the path worn smooth by people with cameras and Hush Puppies. We were approaching the waterfalls for which the upper Tees is popular and on this fine morning the holiday spirit was high. A man with his tie loosened and his jacket over his shoulder strolled past us. He looked at Boogie and said, 'Hello dog.'

Hello human being, replied Boogie.

The attraction here is not only the river. The upper Tees is internationally renowned for its wild flowers, counting among its list of rarities the spring gentian, the Teesdale violet and the pink-flowered primrose. For years enthusiasts have speculated as to why Teesdale should be home for such a range. The theory is that while the rest of post-ice-age Britain was being put in the shade by forests, this area retained a carpet-like tundra. Teesdale became a bright oasis of grassland and its plants were able to survive, then harden, and ultimately become resistant to changes in climate.

We came to the falls at Low Force where The Tees danced down a set of steps. Nearby there was an Information Centre and I was drawn inside by the smell of fresh coffee. I found a fact sheet with drawings of the flora that I might see, and it was an easy decision to opt for an easy day, to just meander upstream looking at flowers.

I asked the woman in the Centre where I should look to find something special and she replied, 'The car park is a good place to start.'

So I wandered round the car park staring at the ground for something I could identify. I recognised a Ford Escort, and a Peugeot 305 estate with an 'I Stop for Dogs' sticker in the window, but of the spring gentian there was no sign. When a man sitting in his car reading the paper asked, 'Lost your car keys?' I gave up and walked back to the river. There, in an open meadow, I discovered that wild flowers are far more enjoyable if you lie down gently among them with a piece of grass in your teeth and try not to crush anything too important.

I read another chunk of *Wuthering Heights* and immediately started to yawn. I thought: this is what walking the Pennine Way is all about: buttercups and sunshine and a novel and no walking.

A family walked along the path and sat down for a picnic very close to me. They looked at me as if to say, 'Is anyone sitting here?' I watched them out of the corner of my book – a very well organised family. Kids were given paper plates and plastic forks, everything was wrapped neatly in cling film. I thought of picnics in my own family, when, as soon as someone mentions the word, Catherine runs into the kitchen and spends hours making devilled eggs so that no-one leaves the house until tea time and the picnic is eaten in the dark. It was something her own mother did and something that our children will do. The compulsion to make devilled eggs at times of excitement is in their genes.

Now the jumbo packet of crisps came out. The kids offered Boogie a handful and he was over there in a flash, oozing social skills. The kids even offered me some and I sat by them and mused, 'why do you think salt and vinegar crisps are in a green packet and cheese and onion are in a blue?'

The father smiled at me. The mother looked away.

'I mean I'd have thought it would have been the other way round,' I went on. 'Doesn't salt and vinegar conjure up blue to you, and cheese and onion green?'

The father had stopped chewing now. He told his children to leave Boogie alone. He said, 'Nice spot this isn't it? Nice waterfall.'

'I wonder who decides what colour crisp packets are?' I said earnestly.

'Walking, are you?' He wasn't looking at me now.

'Yes I am.'

'On your own?'

'Oh yes.'

'How long you been going?'

'Getting on for two weeks now.'

He nodded and started to talk to his wife about something very personal such as what colour carpet they should choose for their extension.

The falls at Low Force were pretty enough but they were just a warm-up for the main event at High Force, and like all good waterfalls you could hear this one before you could see it. A deep well-fed roar grew to a crescendo as you wound your way through scrub to the edge of the gorge and there it was ahead, a beer-brown, foaming torrent, throwing itself over its whinstone cliff into an icy plunge pool seventy feet below.

A small crowd was standing around the lip, taking pictures, holding tightly on to children. They stood as near to the edge as they dared, filled their faces with the blast of air and noise, and licked the spray from their lips.

They looked full of respect, the way people do when they're presented with natural beauty. You could see them trying to concentrate. They shook their heads in awe. They were trying to feel that special feeling that they knew they were supposed to feel in front of spectacles like this, but couldn't quite tune into; the one they'd driven all the way out here to feel, for God's sake, and they weren't going back till they'd felt it. Most stood there for about ten minutes, then went back to the car park to have their picnic with the radio on.

I pressed on, and within fifty yards the sound of the torrent had gone and a big ugly quarry grabbed all the attention. Looking back at the falls you would never have known they were there.

'A fridge freezer went over High Force last winter,' said the lad I met further upstream.

The image of a fridge freezer plunging seventy foot over a waterfall was a striking one. I imagined some dare-devil inside going over for a stunt, but no such thing, the freezer had been carried away in floods.

'The whole valley was under water. Bridges went down. The river was so high no rocks showed at High Force. It was just a sheet.'

He was mending a fence that had also been washed down in the flood. Debris left behind by the high water mark was still enmeshed on it: plastic bags, smashed wood, all sorts of farmyard detritus. 'That wall was washed away as well,' he said, indicating a pile of rubble.

The land around the river had flattened by this point. The hills were set back, and in the sunshine the river babbled and looked gentle and incapable of violence. Yet here were horror stories of an uncontrollable piece of water that knocked down structures and threatened life.

'I've lived here twenty-five years,' said a fisherman further up the bank, 'and I've never seen floods like them. A fridge freezer went over High Force you know.'

The fridge freezer featured in everyone's story. Maybe it would go down in folklore and every year the scene would be re-enacted. An empty fridge freezer would be sent off down river to appease the flood gods. Or each summer there would be a fridge freezer race. Local men would climb inside and paddle downstream to impress local maidens.

This was Forrest-in-Teesdale, and if anywhere could have used some annual event in the pancake race, cheese rolling, tar barrel burning mould, then this was the place. All these villages along the upper Tees had lost their hearts a hundred years ago when the lead mining declined, but none of them looked as redundant as Forrest-in-Teesdale. It wasn't really a village. The houses stood in a wide and open valley, windy and exposed, and the way they were scattered to all corners created a strong sense of isolation.

They were also, curiously, all whitewashed. This was by order of Lord Barnard who owned the estate and all the property, and rented it out on the condition that tenants whitewash their house every two years. So the sparse valley was dotted with these brilliant buildings standing out like lighthouses.

Thank goodness for events like the High Force Inn quiz night, a regular Friday evening get-together. 'It's all a bit of a laff,' said the barman, although it seemed to me to be rather more than that. One man arrived shadow-boxing, getting ready for a contest. He wanted to fire his team up, he said, because The Chamber of Commerce from Middleton were entering that evening and they were the team to beat.

'What was the name of Minnie Caldwell's cat in *Coronation St*?' he asked his team-mates as a warm-up.

They were all discussing Jersey potatoes and didn't know Minnie Caldwell had even had a cat.

I ate a jam sponge and custard as the room filled with smoke and trivia. Some men came in and sat down and I knew they were fishermen. Fishermen all look alike.

'We come here once a year,' one said. 'It's become a tradition.'

'Is that jam sponge?' asked the other. 'I think I'll have one of them.'

'For which football club was Charlie George the darling in 1971?' asked the quizmaster, and thirty heads went down to confer.

'Arsenal,' shouted one of the fishermen, and thirty heads yelled at him to shutup.

'Is there much in the river here?' I asked the fishermen.

'There's nice salmon, thank you very much,' said one. 'It wasn't many years ago they wouldn't even come near the estuary because of the pollution, but now. . . .'

His mate said, 'We can't catch 'em though, 'cos we haven't got a licence.'

I asked him what they did if they caught one by accident. He sniggered and said, 'Put red spots on it with a felt tip and call it a trout.'

'How do you spell Bamber Gascoigne?' asked the quizmaster.

'Who gives a shit?' said the fisherman.

I left as the light began to fade and walked further up the river to find another place to camp. The whitewashed houses now glowed in the dusk. It was a scene out of pioneer country and I was pitching my tent and boiling up tea, searching for a rain cloud. But the stars were coming out again. I had this image of the heavens suffering retention, fit to burst under the strain. Sometime soon they would be unable to resist the urge and get up in the middle of the night to go, and the result would be a deluge like the one last winter. The river would rise and carry me off and I'd go the same way as that fridge freezer.

I climbed into my sleeping bag but was soon disturbed by a rustling outside. I peered out and saw a sheep. 'Hello, sheep,' I said.

It stood there head cocked, eyes fixed. There seemed to have been a sheep in my vision ever since I left home, and I'd never really paid them much attention. Different breeds of course, Swaledale was the most common, but there was also Scotch Blackface, Dalesbreed and Cheviot. I didn't know what this one was, but rather like the wild flowers you didn't need to know the name to admire her.

Boogie stuck his head out too, but ignored the animal. He's never shown any interest in sheep. Like everyone else he regards them as a subspecies. Looking at this old girl though, it seemed unfair that I'd never thought of sheep as anything other than stupid and ugly. She had a smooth black face and grey eyes, a shiny little button nose and dainty feet, a cutey really. I wanted to stroke her and. . . .

I zipped the tent firmly shut. If you're walking the Pennine Way and you start to find sheep attractive, then it's time to get a grip.

I'd been told I would get the best breakfast I'd ever have at Widdybank Farm. But when I got there the following morning I could find no-one about. There was a just a dog barking in a barn and a blue plastic fertilizer bag blowing round the yard. The back door of the house was open and I'm sure if I'd gone in and cooked myself something and left the right money and everything no-one would have minded, but I don't have the cheek to do that sort of thing.

I sat by the river in the warm morning sun and finished some bread and cheese, then pressed on, higher and higher upriver, the land growing wilder, no buildings in sight at all once Widdybank Farm had slipped from view.

The MOD had taken advantage of the isolation and created a firing range on the southerly bank, an unlikely neighbour for the nature reserve on the northern side. And yet here, as in similar sites, wildlife thrived in the company of the military. It seemed nature could cope with bombs and bullets and tanks better than the impact caused by public access.

The river had narrowed to a ribbon of stony water now. As we walked under the cliff at Falcon Flints, at last it gave some indication that its source, high on Cross Fell, was within striking distance. But it was wrong to grow complacent with The Tees. Just as I started to saunter and whistle to myself, we turned a corner and it was all action again as we looked straight up Cauldron Snout.

This was a startling waterfall that seemed to be pouring out of the sky, and it turned The Tees into a frothing monster once again, all push and shove as it charged over another whinstone cliff on five different levels.

The path led us up the slippery rocks by the side of the fall, the spray wetting us, the wind drying us, until we reached the top and were above it all, and there was the view of Teesdale stretching far far back winding slowly east. The Last Wilderness in England is the name the tourist board has given this region, and it was certainly the emptiest part I had ever visited. Although perversely, here at the top of Cauldron Snout, the wildest part of the river had been tamed and dammed and turned into Cow Green reservoir. I'd known this was here but it was still a shock to have the river suddenly and so emphatically blocked off by a huge lump of official concrete.

I stopped and looked at it, thought of a wild animal

caged, then crossed the bridge just below the dam and stepped out of Durham into Cumbria.

I'd known nothing about the Tees until three days before, but now I felt better acquainted with it than most rivers. When it was gone I immediately missed it and the land seemed emptier still.

Birkdale was another remote farm, and like Widdybank there was no-one about, no-one at work in the yard or even a face at a kitchen window, just that ubiquitous blue plastic bag of fertilizer tossed on the wind. It had been the same in most farms I'd been through. The yards were often so inactive you could hear the buildings creak. The only life was the mad bark of sheep dogs locked in a barn aware another dog was on their patch. There were never any people, and the machinery was always idle. I imagined all the farmers inside writing suicide notes.

We joined the Maize Beck, and followed the stream across the moor, the sun beating down now. At last there was a figure walking towards me, the first person I'd seen all day. How was it you could so easily tell the British? Was it the shorts and the skinny legs? Was it the sunburnt face with the peeling nose? Was it the hanky on the head?

There was no doubting this man's credentials as a long distance walker either. He leaned forward at a perfect angle of determination and had his laundry festooning his body and back pack. Socks and pants hanging from his belt, trousers flagging behind him.

'I've always done things back to front,' he said, as he informed me he was walking the Pennine Way from Kirk Yetholm to Edale. 'That's just the kind of person I am, I suppose.'

We sat out of the wind and had lunch in the remains of some crumbled buildings called Moss Shop, the living quarters of what had once been a lead mine. My friend had an ancient rucsack with badges stitched all over it: Whitby, Shrewsbury, Glastonbury. 'You've been about,' I said.

'I got this rucsack on my fourteenth birthday. I've forgotten what all those places look like. Hardly been out of the house for the last fifteen years.'

Like other north-to-southers, this man had already walked the Pennine Way south to north when he was much younger. Now after twenty years of inactivity he'd decided to do it the other way round.

'Why?' I said.

He looked me in the eye. Could he trust me? 'I needed a break,' he said.

'Same here,' I said.

'I found I was sleeping badly. I found myself opening the newspaper and reading the obituaries.'

'I read the obituaries,' I said.

'They're worrying, aren't they?'

'Did you hear about Linford Christie's mother?'

'Yes. Shame.'

I asked him which was the best way to walk the Pennine Way and he said, 'I enjoyed south to north because I had someone with me. My mate Jim. We had a riot. Couldn't find anyone to go with me this time. You're lucky, you've got a dog. He's good company I bet. I haven't got a dog. Got a hamster at home. He's not much fun though.'

Lapwings mobbed us. The Maise Beck bubbled by as a heat haze rose from the mud. I had this fleeting image of not stopping at Scotland, of just keeping on going past the finishing post. Or maybe I'd simply turn round when I reached Kirk Yetholm and walk back. Boogie jumped up and looked me straight in the eye. The bloody dog was telepathic.

'Do you want to know what is the worst thing about the Pennine Way?' asked my friend.

'What?'

'Pub grub.'

'You're probably right. It's chips with everything, isn't it?'

'They're compulsory in some places.'

I'd wanted to have a conversation like this for a long time. Here was a man who understood. I said, 'I ordered spaghetti in one place and she put chips and peas on it.'

He shook his head. 'I mean, you wouldn't have it at home, would you?'

I said, 'Carrots have been my big problem.'

'Don't talk to me about carrots.'

'Every one I've eaten since Edale has disintegrated as soon as I put my fork in it. I really don't believe people enjoy their carrots like that. I'm firmly of the opinion that if chefs of Great Britain cooked carrots *al dente*, then people would respond positively. Imagine it. Nationwide, mushy carrots would be a thing of the past. You could go into a restaurant and confidently . . . sorry.'

'That's all right. It's good to hear someone speaking their mind about carrots.'

'I just like my carrots firm.'

'I understand,' he said.

'A bit crunchy.'

We moved on to how annoying those little sachets of tomato and tartare sauce are. Then on to puddings. I said, 'On the whole puddings on the Pennine Way have been very good.'

'You're right; the puddings have been very good.'

'You get good puddings in the High Force Hotel,' I said.

'I'll make a note of that. You get good puddings in the Stag in Dufton.'

'I'll try one.'

We parted, knowing we'd never see each other again. I

turned round every so often and I thought how lonely he
looked, walking on his own, getting smaller and smaller.
He waved to me once, and no doubt he thought I too
looked lonely. There had never been time to feel lonely
on this trip though. The path was forever throwing up
surprises, and it was about to throw up the biggest surprise
of them all: High Cup.

You'd think any walker on the Pennine Way would
be prepared for High Cup. All the guide books detail
it at length. Photographers love it — it makes a stunning
picture. And of course all walkers talk about it. 'It's
England's Grand Canyon,' said one American, getting a
bit carried away.

Such a build-up is often hard to live up to. But nothing
can spoil or even properly prepare you for High Cup,
particularly if you come at it from the east as most Pennine
Way walkers do. It's the most stunning and memorable
view on the whole walk and, as with the waterfalls on
the Tees, its impact is hugely increased by the complete
lack of warning. You walk into it the way you would a
surprise party.

The moor flattens slightly and there's more sky, but
you're thinking about something else entirely, like the
toffee pudding you're going to have in the Stag in Dufton.
Then the path ends abruptly and you're standing on a rim
with the ground falling away sharply ahead of you, dragging
the senses with it.

The spectacular view ahead is like a basin with one open
end, the sides rimmed with rocky columns that give way
to smooth and steep flanks. The slopes tumble down down
and further down to a river that runs through the valley
like a crack in the china.

Then at the far end everything spills out in a blaze of
green into the Vale of Eden, and there are the Lakeland
fells rising beyond in smoky cloud. It's a view that makes

your whole body beat faster. It's like a glimpse of a bright
and beautiful future.

And it was there, on this breathtaking edge, two weeks
into my journey, that I realised I could do no wrong on
the Pennine Way. It was my destiny to stride along this
soggy backbone of England and not get wet once. Up on
High Cup Nick at four o'clock on a Sunday afternoon I
tasted immortality.

I stood there for ten minutes before I came to. A bird
of prey swooped through the acres of air from one side
of the bowl to the other, soaring and sinking, perfectly
framed. Boogie looked perfectly framed too, sitting on the
cliff staring into space. I fancied that these last few nights
in the wild had touched a nerve in him, and now, faced
with this display, he was responding to his instincts at last.
He studied the valley bottom closely with a look that said:
a dog would have room to move in these parts, put down
roots, meet a bitch, raise a family.

I walked slowly round the rim. In the presence of
something as impressive as this I felt I should be behaving
with more reverence, be doing more than just looking. I
should sit and paint it, or eulogise it in a poem. I should
look into its depths and find the solution to some eternal
puzzle. I should depart a more noble person.

Another couple of walkers reached the edge and pulled
up in awe. I left them alone and began my descent into
Dufton. I'd had the show all to myself, and they deserved
the same.

6. Love and Hadrian's Wall

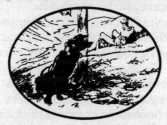

For the next three days I walked with the wind and the sun behind me, head up, hat on, striding over obstacles like Cross Fell with the equanimity of a man plucked out of the crowd to walk the Pennine Way and not get wet once.

The days grew warmer and more sunny. Dark clouds belonged to another country. I stopped looking in the corners of the sky. I developed brown arms and knees. My eyelashes went blond. I began to carry more water than food. Boogie walked with his tongue wrapped round his neck.

I started early in the mornings, then stopped in the afternoons and took my boots off and plunged my feet steaming into a stream. I lay back and fantasised what I'd do if I won the lottery or picked out the £10,000 winner's token from a packet of Walker's crisps, and no matter where these fantasies took me they always brought me back to a patch of cool grass in the Pennines with my boots off and my feet in a stream. There was nowhere I wanted to be more.

The evenings were spent in search of well cooked carrots and good puddings, like the one I almost had in one place, as sleepy a village as you could wish to find: a pub and a post office, a parish notice board and a ring of terracotta-coloured houses round a green. It appeared inert and unexcitable and you couldn't imagine it ever

being any different, even when The Fells Fryer came to
town as advertised on a Tuesday evening, and served fish
and chips from outside the phone box.

And yet the local publican was telling me a different
story. He'd been rushed off his feet all day he said, and his
staff weren't coping. 'We've had a terrible time. We had a
coach party in this afternoon. And this hot weather. . . .'

He seemed to have lots of time to chat even though his
staff were pulling their hair out behind him.

'They were booked in at four o'clock for teas. Well,
only three of them had tea, the rest wanted beer . . .
and meals!'

He hadn't recovered from this outrage. The audacity of
someone coming in and ordering a meal at four o'clock
in the afternoon had been too much to bear. I tried to
calm him down, told him how pretty the village and his
pub were and how undiscovered this whole area seemed to
me, and he said, 'Exactly, we're undiscovered. We want
tourism here, but we don't want it like the Lakes.'

Those debauched Lakes where people frequently asked
for meals at four o'clock.

'I mean if we served meals all day, we'd never have any
time off, would we?'

I ordered a toffee pudding, told him I'd been recom-
mended to try one by a fellow walker. But he put his
fingers to his lips and looked uneasy: 'The chef's a bit on
edge. I don't want to upset him.'

At that point the chef emerged from the kitchen carrying
a plate. 'Haddock and chips,' he announced.

No-one claimed it. The publican said, 'I don't think any-
one ordered that, chef,' and that did it. The chef marched
back to the kitchen and slammed the door. The publican's
wife went back to try to mediate but there were shouts and
the clatter of plates and the publican looked at me and said
quietly: 'I should hang on for your toffee pudding.'

The nights were cool and clear and I spent them camping by streams. Having taken care of Boogie's dental hygiene I turned my attention to his grooming. I washed all the muck off. I combed out his coat. I searched his belly and armpits for tics. I was sure that any day now the complete dog would emerge. He would shed the skin of a baggy-eyed downbeat with no pride in his appearance, and blossom into one of those statuesque black retrievers, head up, shoulders back, mouth open ready to catch a falling duck.

When it got dark I'd build a campfire, boil up rosehip tea and read. I'd abandoned *Wuthering Heights* for local newspapers where the stories were a constant source of wonder: VILLAGE IN DOG FOULING CAMPAIGN. LOCAL MAN FINDS WALLET LOST 20 YEARS AGO. SHOE SHOP BURGLED: NOTHING STOLEN. SHEEP FARMER SHOOTS HIMSELF.

Having plunged down the path rose out like a roller-coaster and this time reached for the summits. There were four peaks to be climbed in one morning, culminating in the highest point in the Pennines, Cross Fell at 2930 feet.

I bought a pie in Dufton post office and dallied on the village green, preparing myself for the climb. A woman walked across with the papers under her arm. She saw Boogie snapping at a fly and said, 'We used to have a dog who did that. But then he started to snap at other dogs, and then he snapped at the postman. So we took him to the vet and she said he was showing pathological behaviour.'

'Tell me more,' I said to her.

'She said he had probably been mistreated at some time in his life, suffered some sort of trauma, and this aggression was a sign of his stress surfacing.'

I thought: maybe Boogie is a dog under stress. I'd

assumed he was just a slob, but he was a victim of some trauma and I was misreading the signs. This snapping at flies was a cry for help.

'What did you do with your dog?' I asked.

'We thought about a course of therapy but in the end we had him castrated.'

Beside me Boogie stopped snapping at the fly and swallowed audibly, then grabbed me by the sleeve and dragged me out of town.

I walked towards Knock Pike trying to ignore the range of peaks to the north. I was happy to stay down here in the Vale of Eden, in the kind of farmland you saw in yoghurt commercials. Just the name was enough to inspire warmth and succour. Why leave the Vale of Eden for Cross Fell?

The path followed tractor lanes, never detouring round a farmyard if it could possibly go straight through it. Why this was, I never could understand. At one point the P.W. signpost seemed to point in through the back door of a farmhouse. 'Excuse me, is this the Pennine Way?' 'Yes, go straight through the kitchen, turn left through the living room, into the study and out through the sun lounge.' 'Thank you. Lovely day for it.'

As the path rose, there were the Cumbrian Mountains, simmering in the haze to the west. They were higher than the Pennines but they looked like rogues. The hills ahead had the baldness of wise old masters, the round shoulders of a watershed. They really looked like the roof of England.

We climbed Knock Pike to the cairn of stones known as Knock Old Man. Then there was Great Dun Fell ahead, with the golf ball of a radar station teed-up on top, having the sort of presence only a radar station can have.

Up and over Little Dun Fell and down to Teeshead, just a soggy patch in the ground, but far to the east the upper Tees was waving like an old friend. From there Cross Fell loomed. It was a summit I'd seen in pictures and on every occasion it had been covered in cloud; reference always made to the fact that up here was recorded the highest wind speed ever in Great Britain, 106 miles per hour.

Today of course it was perfectly visible, but that just let me see what a miserable old git of a hill it was. Stone cairns resembling a line of grim reapers marked the route to the top.

You could only be impressed by the desolation of it all. Nothing lived up here but moss, and that clung on by its fingernails. We trudged on and on, leaning into the wind, the curve of the hill so slight it was hard to judge where the actual apex was. But then Boogie's ears slapped against his face. The day that had been breathless down below was suddenly like being out on deck. The strength of the gale became so great it knocked me sideways, and then I knew we were at the top as the panorama opened and the view became endless.

To the west I could see America, and there was Norway out to the east. There were the Straits of Gibraltar and the Atlas Mountains to the south, and to the north I could make out Kirk Yetholm and The Border Hotel, and my pint of bitter and lasagne and chips waiting for me at the end of the Pennine Way.

A rough, cruciform windbreak of stones had been put together on the summit. I huddled in it and tried to get my stove going, but the wind was too strong, so after a brief rest we followed the track that wound down the northern slope, The Corpse Road – literally a road used to carry corpses from the outlying villages for burial in consecrated ground. The path was as empty as the hills but I fancied I could see a line of souls.

What I could see for sure was a cabin. This was marked on the map as Greg's Hut mountain refuge, so I made straight for it. I wanted to sit inside four walls and brew up. This gale felt like it was bruising me.

As I neared the door I thought I heard a conversation but inside there was no-one, just a room with a few metal beds, a fireplace, and a sign asking visitors to keep the door closed to stop sheep coming in.

Greg's Hut was once a bothy used by miners, in the days when this hillside was riddled with lead workings. Each Monday morning the miners would leave their families in the villages and troop up to the hills to work for the week. On a notice board was an account of a visit by a journalist of the day:

> This house consists of two rooms, and the outer one is a blacksmith's forge (near to which is a stream of running water), a large cupboard which on my visit contained tea, coffee, bacon, bread and even jam. In the inner room are two or three beds, miner's clothing – trousers, stockings and strong heavy boots.

Lead mining, the oldest Pennine industry, had grown up, flourished and died in these hills. 120 years ago, 2000 men were employed, and the villages and surrounding towns were busy, prosperous places. All that remains now is piles of rubble on the empty fells and dark holes in the ground through which the wind whistles. There must be worse places to work in the world but it's hard to imagine them.

I made some tea while the wind howled and rattled the windows. Boogie had been jumpy all morning, unsettled by the thought of castration. Now his ears pricked and he barked and backed against the wall with his legs crossed, as the sound of someone singing came from outside. 'Waterloo. Couldn't escape if I wanted to. Waterloo, finally facing. . . .'

The door scraped open and in came a man wearing headphones and mumbling, 'The history book on the shelf, is always. . . .'

He saw me and stopped singing. We greeted each other in classic hikers' style.

'Blowy out there,' he said.

'Blowy all right,' I replied.

'They're playing hits of the seventies on the radio.'

'Yes.'

'I was just singing. Abba.'

'Yes.'

'Tea. That's a good idea,' he said and pulled out a stove.

'Have some of mine.'

'Thankyou. Would you like a Jacob's Cream Cracker?'

'Just the job.'

He eyed Boogie. 'I was thinking of bringing my dog. But I was frightened I might have to carry him. I listen to the radio instead. The cricket. It's the lunch interval at the moment. That's why I'm listening to hits of the seventies.'

His name was Pete and he was walking the Pennine Way. He said he'd done most of it when he was nineteen, but had had to pack up through injury. Twenty-five years on he was having a second attempt.

'I stumbled jumping across a stream, very near to here. I twisted my knee and that was that.'

He had with him the diary which he'd kept on that first attempt. It was an account of the path in the sixties, not long after it had opened.

'I spent most nights sleeping in farmers' barns. They couldn't understand what I wanted to walk all that way for, but they always let me sleep somewhere.'

He read his old diary: 'it says here that I arrived at Sleightholme Farm one dark night and the farmer let me sleep in the long shed with his prize sheep. I had dry straw and a sack as a blanket and then the farmer's wife brought supper of fruit cake and tarts, biscuits and a huge pot of tea. Another time the farmer let me sleep in his hay loft for two shillings. I didn't take my boots off for four days once.'

He smiled ruefully. 'I've stayed in nice bed-and-breakfasts and taken my boots off every night this time.'

I walked with him down towards the village of Garrigill as the path curved round the back of all the fells we'd climbed that day. The wind dropped and it grew warm again. We reached a stream which was so dry it was hardly noticeable, but Pete stopped and said, 'I think this is it. This is the place I sprained my knee.'

There was hardly any water in it. You didn't have to jump it to cross.

'It was full then, of course,' said Pete. 'You had to leap over or get your feet wet.'

He looked misty-eyed as he remembered the nineteen-year-old lad leaping over streams. He sprang over the gap. 'Careful,' I said. 'Don't do it again.'

He laughed. 'Silly thing to do really,' and he jumped back again.

I asked if this time was very different from the previous, and he said, 'Navigation was a lot harder then, that's for sure. The path was popular but it hadn't been walked enough to make a definite line. The signposts were irregular as well. And there were none of these walkways made of stone slabs. You spent the day up to your elbows in peat.'

'Was it better then or now?'

'Now,' he said, and then in a whisper, in case someone from the Ramblers' Association overheard, 'I like stone slabs.'

'So do I,' I admitted.

'You can't go getting sentimental over things like peat bogs.'

'No.'

We walked further down the track and when we got to another stream he said, 'actually I was wrong back there. This is where I sprained my knee.'

A farmer let me camp in a field in Garrigill that night, by the South Tyne river. There were three other tents. I thought: songs by the camp fire, Pennine Way tales.

I found the other campers in the pub. Two sweaty men, with blotchy faces and red hairy legs in khaki shorts. And two women, blonde, brown and lovely, dressed in clothes that hung gracefully to their bodies. I ordered lasagne and chips and sat down opposite them.

'They're all crap these days,' said one of the men in a Midlands accent. He was eating something with custard on.

'What about *Absolutely Fabulous*?' one of the women responded in a northern European accent. She had a plate of food in front of her which she'd hardly touched.

'First series was all right. The second was dreadful,' said the other man, and peeled a lump of skin off his sunburnt neck. I remembered an American friend saying once: Englishmen are all right, but you can't take them to the beach.

'We get *Absolutely Fabulous* in Holland,' said the woman, who was more than likely Dutch.

Television as detente. You could go most places in the world and meet people these days with a working knowledge of situation comedies past and present. These two likely lads couldn't believe their luck. They'd cornered two Dutch women and all they were having to do to impress them was wheel out old TV titles.

'*Cheers* was my favourite,' said the other Englishman.

'Oh I loved *Cheers*,' said the other Dutch woman. Then she looked out of the window and laughed and I could see what had started the conversation. She could see through the window across the street and into a house where there was a TV on, and there was the unmistakable sight of John Cleese as Basil Fawlty. It was staggering to think you could recognise a TV programme through two windows and across a street.

'It's the one about the Germans,' she said. 'I saw in the paper. Don't mention the war.' They all laughed and then fell silent as they tried to watch it.

One of the women patted Boogie and gave him the remains of her pâté and toast to stop him drooling over her sandals. When I told her we were walking the Pennine Way she just said, 'You British and your dogs,' and shook her head pitifully.

They didn't want my company, or at least the two men didn't. They'd dreamed that the Pennine Way was going to be a long line of pretty Dutch women but never in their hearts had they really believed it. Now that it was really happening they weren't going to let a third party muscle in.

As I left the pub one of the men said, 'Do you get *Mr Bean* in Holland?'

'Oh I love *Mr Bean*,' said a Dutchwoman.

'There are lots of people like Mr Bean in England,' said the other one, and the men sort of laughed.

They didn't stand a chance.

I was away the next morning before there was any sound from the other tents. It was a grey day with low cloud. A man in the village emptied his dustbin and said, 'Don't worry, it'll clear up.'

But I wasn't worried; I knew it wouldn't rain. And

anyway I had the feeling all Mondays in Garrigill started off like this, as if in remembrance of days past when the lead workers got up at dawn, packed a bag and headed off up to Greg's Hut. It was hard to imagine this little grey village full of activity. It looked so content in its retirement. There was a very attractive house in the middle of the green with stairs going up the outside, suggesting one of those farms where the residents lived on the top floor and cattle were kept underneath to warm the house. 'It's a holiday home now,' said the man with the dustbin. 'You wouldn't get anyone local living in that. There's no garden. Where are you going to grow your veg?' Where indeed?

The morning stayed humid and misty but there were no views on this stretch into the town of Alston and so I missed nothing. The path followed the South Tyne river through woodland for most of the way.

The first feature of the day was a tip. Not your everyday sort of tip though, this was rural rubbish: tractor shells, old railway carriages and lumps of agricultural scrap. And there were rabbits running round and chickens lived there and it didn't smell, so it couldn't really be called unpleasant. I walked past thinking: a long distance path needs a few rubbish tips to give it some credibility.

We marched the four miles into Alston, Boogie now negotiating stiles with ease. It was hard to remember how two weeks previously he would stop and wait for me to throw him over. Now he took them at a run as if he enjoyed them and he was over them with a bound.

Alston had been the centre of the lead mining industry and its legacy was a cobbled high street from which alleys and lanes led off and tied themselves in knots. It was a delightful town where you found yourself forever peering round corners. The Pennine Way isn't known as a shopping holiday, but Alston is the nearest it comes to one. Down every alley you'll find some sort of curious shop, such as the grocers that has a collection of antique bottles for sale.

I came across a pottery shop called Pots For The Pennine Landscape. I stood outside with Boogie and peered in, and the potter peered out and thought to herself: he's not coming in here with that dog, is he? Oh God, he is!

I tied Boogie to the door and tiptoed round. All the pottery had been inspired by the hills, hills which at a glance appeared bleak and amorphous, and yet these pots were so striking. They had captured shades and hues that I would never have believed were up there had I not walked the moors. They were interwoven with strands of pink, purple, crimson and plum, pale browns that blended into pale blues. These were the underlying colours of the Pennines.

'It looks different every time I go up there,' said the potter. Syl Marco was her name and she talked about how the moors changed at different times of the day and the year, and in different weathers. I saw one plate in blue and pale yellow and grey, and it immediately brought back the colours of that warm and clear afternoon when I'd climbed out of Upper Teesdale.

It was Catherine's birthday soon and I'd been looking to buy her something like this. I struggled with the thought of walking the Pennine Way with a large, fragile and valuable pot banging about in my back pack, but Syl said she could wrap one and post it for me. I chose a blue-, grey-and pearl-coloured vase. 'It'll be home before you will,' she said.

Outside a Blue Circle cement truck groaned its way up the cobbled street. The driver looked apologetic, like a giant trying to creep through the town and not tread on anything. The charm of a place like Alston is that it's untouched by the traffic planner, but you sensed it was just a matter of time. There was already a Bohemian spirit here. It looked unpretentious and lived-in but it wouldn't take much for a Hebden Bridge to spring up.

I sat outside the station café, surrounded by railway memorabilia as the sun burst through. A young couple in leathers sat nearby. He was blowing his nose; she was reading yesterday's newspaper. He said, 'Bloody warmest week of the year and I've got a cold.' He wanted to blame someone.

I asked them what they did in Alston. 'Nothing,' he said, and blew his nose again. She put her paper down and said she was a babysitter. She got work five nights of the week. Some nights she got double-booked and she contracted out. She was like an agent. '£1.50 an hour for watching telly,' she said. 'It's a good job.'

It was also very enterprising. In small market towns like this throughout the country teenagers complained of nothing to do in the evening, and ended up sitting on railings in the centre of town, or taking cans of lager into the kids' playgrounds. As soon as these two could drive, they planned to go and live in Newcastle and never come back.

'I hate living here,' he said, but his cold had turned him into a misery and he hated everything. I asked him what Hadrian's Wall was like and he said, 'Seen one wall, seen 'em all.'

Now he was taking his cold out on the Roman Emperor Hadrian, and this was unfair. I'd seen a lot of walls on this walk and I was damn sure Hadrian's was going to be something different.

It was the next attraction on the Pennine Way, and after Alston, just knowing it was within striking distance made me want to quicken my pace. It lay directly north and when I discovered that there was a disused railway line that led to a town just below the Wall I decided to follow it. The Pennine Way was heading in the same direction along a parallel route, but walking an old railway line felt like a pleasant change, and then when I saw the town that the line led to was called Haltwhistle, it seemed like the only route to take. I got a kick out of walking somewhere just because I liked the name.

Someone should write a song about Haltwhistle, I thought, as I set off from platform one. If Haltwhistle was in America it would have had half a dozen tunes singing its praises. *Only 24 Hours From Haltwhistle. Haltwhistle, Haltwhistle One Hell of a Town.* British towns never got that sort of treatment and yet on the Pennine Way there had been many placenames worthy of a song: *I Left my Heart on Kinder Scout. Horton in Ribblesdale Wants Me. But I Can't Go Back There. By The Time I Get to Kirk Yetholm.*

A musical version of the Pennine Way, now there was an idea. Imagine the hike over Bleaklow choreographed, or the climb up Fountains Fell put to lyrics. It would be the story of a boy Pennine Way walker meeting a girl Pennine Way walker in Edale. He saves her life on Black Hill. She saves his on Penyghent. He falls for a sheep on Great Shunner Fell but she wins his love back in the flower-filled meadows of Swaledale. They get married at Tan Hill choosing buffet B with the cheese and onion crolines. Imagine the cast of an entire West End stage dressed in Gore-tex.

I followed the railway line ever north, recognising the stage on a long distance trek when the days slip into each other, you catch yourself talking to yourself, and you plod on spending long periods considering items you would normally let drop through the holes in your pocket without a thought. One minute I was considering a Broadway musical, the next I was thinking how big the slugs were on this stretch, great black things with horns.

And following a railway line was like walking along a corridor, like a canal, no need to concentrate, maps and navigation abandoned for the day. Just go with the line as it wound through the South Tyne valley.

Every now and again the river would appear, another one of these great north-eastern rivers with an industrial tradition, but like a puppy here, and the water so clear.

I strode in and out of cuttings not knowing what to expect next. This must have been a fine railway once. It operated for a hundred years but, like everything in these parts, declined with the lead mining, and ultimately closed in 1976. The local council had only recently decided to maintain it as a path. At Lamberly they were even restoring the fabulous viaduct.

I came down to the river here and did some washing and threw some stones for Boogie. Days like this were effortless and had slipped by before I knew it. Ah look, a bench! A shame to pass a bench and not sit on it, and so I sat and looked up at the moors to the west and knew that the Pennine Way was bound to be climbing about up there somewhere, and I felt happy to be down here reading the classified ads in the Alston local paper: *Hamster cage for sale £20, free hamster included. Will deliver.*

It wasn't until the early evening that the line curved to the west over another impressive viaduct and the town of Haltwhistle came into view, spread over a hillside. Just a mile beyond was Hadrian's Wall, and I continued until I was almost in its shadow, then found a farm. I wanted a night inside; I needed a bath.

A woman stopped me as I turned up the drive. She asked, 'Is this the way to the bed and breakfast?' She was German.

Looks like it is, I said to her, and we arrived on the doorstep at the same time. The farmer assumed we were together.

'I'm single,' the German said very firmly.

'So am I,' I said, not quite so firmly as the German but firmly enough.

The farmer's wife made a big fuss of Boogie. 'Has he got a blanket? I'll get him a blanket. Would he like some warm milk? Has he eaten? 'Cos I've got lots of dog food. Leave him with me. I want him to meet Grace.'

She led him into the kitchen where a dog half his size lay by the Aga. As she stood up, though, I checked myself. Grace was a bull terrier. Boogie stepped back as well, looked at me with a 'that's one of those isn't it. The ones that keep getting in the paper.'

But the woman was saying. 'Oh don't worry about Grace. She's not at all aggressive.'

Grace looked at her with an 'oh yes I am, I'm horribly aggressive!'

'You know what she likes doing most of all. Lying on the couch having her tummy tickled and listening to Paul McCartney on the stereo.'

Grace sidled over to Boogie. Boogie positioned himself at my side so that with one bound he could be in my pocket. Grace stuffed her nose between his legs and he didn't dare move.

'They've hit it off, look,' said the farmer's wife. 'Why doesn't he come and sit on the couch?

Boogie looked at me with a 'Don't leave me with this animal. I'm frightened. Please. They kill after they mate.'

I went to find the bathroom, and there was the German woman coming out of her door. I said to her, 'Are you going to have a bath?' and she stared at me briefly, then went back into her room. I heard the lock turn.

I drew a deep bath and lay there looking at the photos on the wall. This was a nice place to stay; these looked like good people. There was the farmer pinning a first prize rosette on a cow at some agricultural show. There was his wife riding a horse over jumps. They felt like distant relations and these were scenes that I should recognise.

I went to fetch Boogie to go out for something to eat,

but from the kitchen I could hear the sound of Paul McCartney. I didn't want to interrupt anything, so I left him and strolled down to the pub.

The German woman was already sitting there struggling with a Cumberland sausage. 'Did you have a nice bath?' she asked

'Very nice. There was some Batman bubble bath.'

'I could not have a bath. The house is too cold.'

Her name was Ursula and she didn't look very happy. She was walking the Pennine Way, but she was taking it very slowly – more than three weeks to get this far – and she was doing it in style. She stayed at the best, most expensive places she could find.

'I like to have my own bathroom. I like to have my own toilet. I like to stay at places that have central heating and three crowns from the English Tourist Board.'

'The Pennine Way can be anything you want it to be,' I said.

'I want it to be comfortable.'

She'd started with a friend. But the friend had dropped out.

'She went to stay at a nice hotel in the Lake District,' she said, through gritted teeth.

I offered her a drink and she asked for cider, and for the rest of the evening whenever her glass was empty she passed it to me to refill. Each time I went to the bar I imagined the barman was winking at me: that's the way; get her drunk on cider. Ha Ha.

'Does your dog like Cumberland sausage?' asked Ursula.

'I'm sure he does,' I replied, and she wrapped it up in a napkin and handed it to me, then she went and ordered a lasagne and when that came she didn't eat that either. 'Does your dog like lasagne?' she asked.

'Loves it,' I said, and she wrapped that up too. I asked

her if she was enjoying the path. She thought about it hard
and then answered: 'Yyes.'

'What do you think of pub grub?'

She seemed to ignore the question. She sat back
and said: 'You know something? I have at least two
holidays a year.'

'That's nice.'

'I have a good job. I'm thirty-two years old and I work
in publicity. I have no dependants. My time and my money
are my own and so I go on holiday a lot.'

'I used to be like that.'

'One holiday I have in the winter, and I do something
very lazy, lie on a beach somewhere hot, tropical. This
year I went to the Caribbean, last year to the Far East. I
went to Australia one year, to the Barrier Reef.'

'I've always wanted to go there.'

'The other holiday I do something adventurous, some-
thing that will get me fit. I have trekked into the jungle
in Peru. I have gone sledging above the Arctic Circle. I
have climbed a mountain in Africa.'

'Wonderful.'

'And you know something?'

'What?'

'On all my travels, in all the countries I have been to, I
have never come across anything so ugly as Pub Grub.'

'I see.'

'It's crap.'

'You do speak good English.'

'There is only one thing as strange as Pub Grub.'

'What's that?'

'A Full English.'

'A Full English Breakfast?'

'That's him. Black pudding is obscene.'

'Bed and Breakfasts are good though, aren't they?' I said
cheerfully. 'You do get to meet the local people.'

She took a deep breath: 'I stayed at one Bed and
Breakfast in Hebden Bridge where the man parked his
motorbike in the living room.'

'Parking is very bad in Hebden Bridge.'

'Then in the village of Gargrave the lady played Barry
Manilow records until midnight.'

'The one tonight is very nice though, isn't it?'

'It's cold.'

I got another drink. The barman was definitely winking
at me. When I got back to the table Ursula looked even
more miserable, so I asked, 'What do you think about
the comedy on TV in England?' And she brightened up
immediately.

'Oh I love *Mr Bean*,' she laughed, threw her head back
and took her coat off.

We walked back to the house. The cider had got her in a
much better mood, and the long talk we had had about
English situation comedies had made her laugh. She had
lost her serious face and she was giggling the way those
Dutch women had the night before. My stomach tightened
as the evening took on sexual potential.

Ursula said, 'You know what my ambition is while I
am in England?'

'What?'

'I want to find a café that will serve me a cup of tea after
five o'clock in the afternoon.'

I laughed. 'Good luck.'

When we got to the front door I fumbled with the key
and she said, 'I hope I will be warm enough tonight.'

'Oh, I'm sure you will. This is a warm spell we're having,
you know.'

'Will you be warm enough?'

'Oh, I'll be warm enough.'

'You've got your dog, haven't you?'

What she meant by that I didn't know. I'd dig a snow hole before I resorted to cuddling up to Boogie.

We got into the hallway and stood by a picture of the farmer pinning a rosette on a pig, and his wife holding a fruit cake. Ursula looked at me and said, 'I think I'll have an early night.'

'Good idea,' I replied, and we slipped into our rooms.

I lay on my bed with my boots on, thinking: I didn't want to go back to her bedroom. I didn't. But it would have been nice to have been asked.

I suddenly remembered Boogie. I listened for the sound of Paul McCartney but could hear nothing, and I hurried into the kitchen where the farmer and his wife were doing a jigsaw. Grace and Boogie were on the couch, Grace staring into his eyes. Boogie had a look that said: 'honestly, I'm married with three puppies at home.'

'They've been good as gold,' said the farmer. 'I think he's taken a shine to her.'

I took Boogie back to the room. 'You little devil,' I said. 'You've still got it, haven't you? All it took was a bit of fresh air and exercise, and they're like flies round a. . . .'

I tensed as I heard Ursula's door open down the corridor and her feet pad down the hall. But she went past my door and downstairs to the kitchen. I heard her say: 'I am cold.' She was sounding sober and serious again.

'Would you like a hot water bottle?' asked the farmer.

'I would like the central heating on.'

There was no reply to that. The door closed and Ursula padded up the stairs and back to her room. I could just hear the farmer whispering to his wife: 'she wants the central heating on!'

'In July?'

'Aye.'

'Did you tell her we're having a hot spell.'

'Aye.'

'It's ridiculous.'

'That's what I said.'

'What shall we do?'

'I don't know. What do you think?'

'I don't know.'

They were reasonable people. They did their best to make guests comfortable. They offered them three pillows, and a choice of four different sorts of breakfast cereal including muesli; and they loved it when people brought their pets to stay.

All they asked in return was for guests to clean the ring round the bath after them and not to smoke in bed. But now here was someone (from abroad) asking for the central heating on in July.

Some things just weren't done.

After a few minutes the boiler chugged reluctantly into life. Ten minutes later it went off again. I lay there knowing that there was one way to get the heating turned up, get the place humming in fact: just tell them Boogie was feeling a bit chilly.

Hadrian's Wall. A, if not the, highlight of the journey. A special day.

Ursula slept in late and I had breakfast on my own. Our hosts still hadn't recovered from the demands of the previous evening. She said, 'I'm sorry but we had to turn the boiler on last night.'

'Yes I heard.'

'In July! She was cold. . . .' – She mouthed these words with a whisper and cast her eyes upstairs to where Ursula slept in her anorak – '. . . . in July. In a warm spell.'

I got ready to go but when they saw Boogie walk with a stiff leg they refused to let him leave the house. 'He's limping,' said the farmer.

'He does that every morning.'

'He needs a day off.'

'He's fine. It wears off after ten minutes.'

But Boogie looked up at them with his orphaned expression and they insisted he have some hot milk and cereal. Then when they suggested I leave him at the house while I went and looked at Hadrian's Wall on my own, it seemed like a good idea. I wanted to spend some time at the sites and I wanted to visit museums where Boogie wouldn't have been welcomed.

'Grace will be grateful for the company,' said the farmer, and Grace swaggered over to him like Mae West in a cocktail dress.

Another misty morning, a blotting paper day. It might even have rained in the night; the road had a glassy sheen, looked newly painted. The shrouded countryside added to the sense of anticipation. As I walked along the road to the Wall, I peered over each rise, expecting to catch a glimpse of something that would stop me in my tracks.

I passed what looked like a quarry, then came through a small wood, emerging to follow a low stone wall which I expected would join up with Hadrian's at any moment. Then it dawned on me this was Hadrian's. I'd been looking all around for the monster when I'd been standing on its back.

I pulled up in fright, stood back from it, reached out and touched it, expecting to get an electric shock or some frisson at least. I wanted this moment to be memorable, but it wasn't. Because of the mist you couldn't see more than forty yards. The idea that this wall stretched forty miles in each direction was difficult to believe.

The Pennine Way actually followed the line of the Wall eastward from here, but I didn't want to walk it in these conditions, I'd have seen nothing. So I ducked into the Roman Army Museum nearby.

Ten o'clock on a Tuesday morning and I was the only person in there. A woman served me coffee and said, 'It'll lift. It's been like this in the mornings all week.'

I trailed round the exhibits; stared through glass cabinets at the bits of broken pottery, coins, Roman combs, old Roman shoes and battered spearheads. I read Roman recipes. I digested the charts showing the distribution of Roman soldiers over the empire. I pressed all the buttons on the audio visual display and I felt my eyelids droop. A lassitude was creeping over me like a drug. I wanted to climb on that Roman soldier's bed and curl up.

'Still not lifted, has it?' said the woman behind the counter, making me jump.

I had another coffee and wandered round the gift shop. A man in shorts and anorak came in and fingered the gift boxes of shortbread, the preserves in presentation boxes, the Hadrian's Wall fudge. 'I need a gift,' he said. He was American and his glasses had steamed up.

'Can you see the wall yet?' I asked

'No. Socked in still. But I saw it yesterday.'

'Impressed?'

'You bet. It was bigger than I thought it would be.'

That was strange. With monuments as famous as this, most people had seen so many pictures beforehand that when they came to see the real thing, they were disappointed. They always said it looked smaller.

The American said, 'That's what the people in the guest house warned me of. So I prepared myself for something smaller. But I overcompensated and so, although it was smaller than it was in the pictures, it was bigger than I had imagined, and so I wasn't disappointed.'

The doors were flung open and in came a party of school children. They charged up to the ticket machine and overflowed into the gift shop, sending the staff frantic as they rummaged through the Roman rulers and rubbers.

The teachers tried to coral them like cowboys would fifty head of cattle, but the kids were on the stampede. They ran round the museum, pressing all the buttons and aping the models, the boys going to extreme lengths to impress the girls, grabbing spears off displays and impaling class mates for a laugh. The teachers held their heads. They'd kept them on the bus too long. I grabbed my bag and went outside.

The mist was burning away slowly and the wall was more visible now. In some places I could see it had been restored to a height of five feet or more. In others it had been razed and scavenged for the stone and become grassed over. But its course was discernible into the distance and it began to look imperious as it snaked away over the whin sill, that hard, black seam of rock that had first appeared back in Upper Teesdale and had been responsible for the spate of waterfalls. Now it resurfaced, rearing angrily up out of the terrain, a natural site to build a defensive line.

The reasons why the Emperor Hadrian built his wall are debatable. The most obvious one was to form the northern defence of the Roman Empire. It would have been typical of him to initiate such a project. It was reported he was a tidy man and he liked the idea of wrapping his territory up.

But there are also theories that he ordered the wall to be built simply to give his soldiers something to do on this northernmost frontier, where military life was tough and dull, and Rome was a long way away. Certainly the soldiers built it in double quick time, taking just two years to brick off the whole country from coast to coast. You could imagine how these days such an engineering project would produce five years of paperwork before anyone lifted a shovel.

The view was improving by the minute as I followed the wall, gazing north over the cliff of the sill to the land of the Picts, the Barbarians.

At Cawfield Crags was a very well preserved section. They say Hadrian had heard stories of the Great Wall of China, and from here that was what came to mind, a dragon of a wall, bucking and twisting, religiously following the contours of the land, no obstacle too big or awkward for it to climb. The whole panorama was grey and threatening, and if you focused on it you could easily transport yourself back in time to the days when this was a well-armed frontier. You just had to ignore the military jets buzzing around at head height.

Once again the path was the background, just the link-road between attractions. I came down to visit Vindolanda, the site of a garrison. Here was an excellent exhibit that brought the period and the Roman occupation wonderfully to life. They'd even reconstructed a section of wall complete with a watch tower.

And then in the museum there was the most haunting of all the discoveries made in the many years of archaeological excavation on the site: a collection of letters and documents from the time of the Roman occupation that had sunk into a layer of wet clay and had been preserved.

They had been thrown on fires in fact, fires that are thought to have been lit to destroy documents towards the end of the occupation when the garrison was closing down. When the first fragments were found they were obviously charred, and yet there was no evidence of a fire in the immediate vicinity. The assumption was made that they had been blown off a fire, and so the hunt for its site began and went on for years. When finally it was located, no-one was prepared for the wealth of material that was unearthed.

Letters, shopping lists, books, accounts, social diaries; invites to birthday parties; letters from soldiers complaining about food, lack of beer and poor roads. All documents pertaining to ordinary people living ordinary lives, the minutiae of everyday existence in a Roman garrison, and all saved because a Northumberland downpour had put a fire out. It wouldn't have happened this summer.

Back on the Wall, the afternoon was turning hot again and the views were impressive in every direction as the course followed the crest of the whinstone wave and swerved away over the crags past milecastles.

There was water below the wall now – a lake – so that the effect was of walking along a cliff path. This was the area known as Cuddy Crags and was probably the most photographed section of all, the one you see on all the brochures, posters and calendars. It was also accessible from the car parks and attracted all the tourist bus groups.

A group of Americans passed me, dressed in coloured shorts and hats and carrying camcorders. They were exuberant. England was living up to all expectations. As I passed one woman she held out her camera to me and asked me to take a picture of her and her sister. I obliged and then she wanted to take a picture of me. I couldn't understand why on earth she wanted to do this, but she said she was taking pictures of as many English people as she could.

I felt like a native. I could see the picture on the slide projector back home in Ohio with the caption: Englishman walking on Hadrian's Wall.

She asked, 'Where do you live?'

'Derbyshire.'

'I thought you had an accent.'

I backed off before she offered me money to do a clog dance.

That night the farmer and his wife offered me tea and biscuits in their kitchen where they were still poring over their jigsaw. Boogie and Grace were on the couch. She was nibbling his ear. He was watching a blank TV.

'We bought this for the grandson,' said the farmer. 'But it's a thousand pieces. Bit difficult for him.'

So they were doing it themselves. It was an amusing scene – a couple in their fifties doing a jigsaw of an evening – but it was addictive. The jigsaw was an illustrated map of the British Isles and when I saw a piece with a windmill on I could see it was a chunk of East Anglia and I slotted it in place.

'Give us a hand if you like,' said the farmer. 'I'm Jack, by the way. And that's Alice.'

Alice said, 'Can you see half a Scotsman tossing a caber? 'Cos I've got the other half.'

That was the kind of jigsaw it was – cartoon drawings of typical British scenes. As well as a man in a kilt tossing a caber, Scotland was represented by the Loch Ness monster and a cave where Robert the Bruce was hiding. England was depicted the way it was in Ealing comedies or in Disney Films: Robin Hood stood over Nottingham; Stephenson's Rocket steamed out of Darlington; Liverpool was the home of the Beatles.

I asked Jack and Alice where they went on their holidays and Jack said, 'We don't need to go on holiday, not living here.'

And you could almost see their house on this jigsaw, just below the Roman centurion patrolling Hadrian's Wall.

I slotted an oil rig into the North Sea, a castle and a lump of Caerphilly cheese into Wales, some scholars on bicycles into Oxford and Cambridge. Down in Cornwall I found homes for Merlin and King Arthur.

And then there were the Pennines, illustrated by a couple hiking in T-shirts and shorts, and I realised that this was the kind of England I had walked through these last two or three weeks. I'd strode over moors that the Brontës had strode over. I'd passed through dales where James Herriot was king. I'd eaten full English breakfasts until they were coming out of my ears, and all through a summer that had been Battle of Britain blue.

It was all so perfect it was enough to make me feel uneasy, make me long for a world I felt more familiar with. I would have felt more comfortable with a jigsaw where Bradford was depicted by race riots, where Luton had a line of motor industry redundancies, where London was ringed with a traffic jam, and the Pennines were covered by a big black cloud and any hiker was lying face down in a peat bog. The trouble with this walk was that it had shattered all my illusions.

I had a pang of homesickness. I wanted to be in my own kitchen doing a jigsaw with my own family. Now that we'd reached Hadrian's Wall, maybe the journey should end anyway. The Pennines stopped here, so why didn't the Pennine Way? From here the path headed north to climb the Cheviots, for no reason I could see.

I said as much to the farmer, as he looked for a slot for the Loch Ness Monster. 'I feel as though I've done it all,' I said. 'Seems hardly worth walking through the Cheviots.'

He looked at me sternly, pointed the Loch Ness monster at me and said, 'You don't want to go underestimating the Cheviots, bonnie lad. The Cheviots are bastards!'

7. The Bastard Cheviots

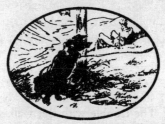

You're up in your attic, sorting through boxes, musty piles containing the litter of your life. You pick your way through the old football programmes, yellowing newspapers, black and white snaps of someone with an embarrassing haircut who could just be you, memorabilia that at a glance brings back moments you thought you'd forgotten.

Because you're having your attic converted, aren't you? The kids are growing up and want more space. You could move, but why not just create another room, put in a dormer window, build another storey; costs a bit but think of it as added value on the house.

Look at that! A train ticket to Rome dated 1973. And there's an old wage slip – £20 for a week's work in the pork pie factory. Which pile does that go on? The keep-it or chuck-it-out. The chuck-it-out is very small; the keep-it is toppling already. Hell, if a wage slip has made the effort and lasted this long, why not keep it for another twenty years.

What's that at the bottom of the box, just under your O-level results? A creased piece of paper, torn out of an exercise book, written in a hand no longer even recognisable as your own. It's a list:

1) Appear on Top of Pops.

2) Cycle a tandem to China picking up hitchhikers.
3) Write a cult novel.

You laugh as you realise these were the ten aims you promised yourself you would achieve by the time you were thirty.

4) Date one of the girls from Abba.
5) Own a Porsche by age twenty-five.
6) Learn to speak German and French.
7) Don't get married until thirty-three.
8) Never become so suburban and middle class as to want to convert your loft into an extra bedroom.
9) Invent something. Anything.

And there, tucked in at number 10, you find it: Walk the Pennine Way.

You shake your head and throw the list on the chuck-it-out pile. They were ambitions from years ago, when you knew nothing. They were ambitions you don't even remember having. But that's not what is unsettling about them. What makes you stop and unfold the bit of paper and run down the list again is the realisation that almost all of them, all those goals, are now beyond you. Face it, you're as likely to learn to speak French now as you are to appear on Top of the Pops, as you are to own a Porsche. Only one of them is still possible: Number 10, Walk Pennine Way.

The screams of the kids filter up through the floorboards. The image of yourself striding along the northern uplands, across the roof of Britain is suddenly very clear. How long is it since you did something like that? Went back to basics, lived off berries, slept rough. So long you've forgotten what it was like. If you told people you were going to walk the Pennine Way now they'd just laugh.

A huge idea enters your head. Why not show them what you're really made of? Think what your mates would say down the pub: 'Have you heard about Frank? He just upped and went. Spontaneous decision. One minute he was a slob, the next he was walking to Scotland. You've got to hand it to the bloke.'

And you could do it. 'Course you could. You're still fit – well, fittish. It's just a question of walking, and middle-aged men are better at this sort of thing than younger men. They can pace themselves better. They're better disciplined. It would do you the world of good too. Lose some weight. You've been saying you're going to join that gym, why not get some proper exercise. Pit yourself against the elements. Go down now and announce it: 'I've decided to walk the Pennine Way. . . .'

This scenario, or a variation on it, was actually how most of the walkers I'd met had ended up on the path to Kirk Yetholm, particularly the male ones, particularly the middle-aged male ones. That was how the man I met sitting on a log in the Wark Forest had ended up there. He really had found a list up in his attic and now he was going to 'prove he could still do it'.

This was a surprise, because if I'd been asked to describe the typical Pennine Way walker before I left, I would have drawn a young lad, nutbrown, well-equipped, walking with his mate, doing it in two weeks, not conscious of the time they had, and doing it too quickly.

But this had never been the case. The typical Pennine Way walker was this man tucking into his banana sandwiches, a forty-five-year-old with a peeling nose, sitting on the rucsack he'd been given on his twelfth birthday, wearing shorts that nicely displayed an incipient varicose vein, and always a glint in his eye, a glint that said, I don't

believe it! I'm actually walking the Pennine Way and loving
every minute of it.

And they all seemed to be doing the path 'before it got
too late', as if they would lose the use of their legs the
minute they reached Kirk Yetholm or Edale. This man had
only been going three days – he was a north to souther –
but he was already a changed person.

'I'm beginning to realise something has been missing in
my life over the last twenty-five years,' he said.

'What do you do?' I asked.

'I work for a company that sells doors.'

'Doors . . . as in . . . doors?'

'Yes, doors. It's a good business. People need doors.
Have a guess how many doors the average house has.'

'I don't know. Ten?'

'Fifteen.'

'Really.'

'See, people underestimate doors. They take doors for
granted.'

'Like windows,' I said.

'Exactly. People take windows for granted too. We used
to do windows as a matter of interest. Windows and doors.
But then we decided to specialise in doors.'

He quizzed me about the path ahead. But I found I
couldn't tell him much. I'd taken so many detours there
were chunks of the Pennine Way I'd missed out. I just
told him to notice how the streams, that were known on
this part of the map as burns and sikes, would change to
becks in Yorkshire, and how he'd know when he got to
Edale, because there they were called cloughs.

He was keen to get moving, the way people are when
they've just started a long journey. I watched him stride
away with the enthusiasm of a little boy and I thought:
he's going to get home and discover that that list of
ambitions he found in the attic isn't his, it's his brother's

or someone's, but by then it'll be too late, he'll have been Pennine Wayed.

No doubt walking the Pennine Way once figured high on Boogie's list of ambitions, somewhere between winning Best Mongrel at Crufts, and playing understudy to Lassie. Now with just three days to go to the Scottish border, it looked as though he was about to realise his goal. He wouldn't be the first dog to walk the Pennine Way, but he would probably be the least well-bred.

We were walking to Bellingham, somewhere I'd visited once before. I'd spent the day at the Bellingham Show about ten years ago, and then had a wild evening afterwards. It seemed the whole showground, including some of the animals, had crammed into a little pub in the village called the Fox and Hounds. At closing time the landlady locked the door but never asked anyone if they wanted to leave first. I met an Italian who had been passing on a motorcycle and had stuck his head in to ask directions. He was handed a whisky, given a kiss by a woman who'd won first prize for her Bakewell Tart, and that was as far as he got for the night.

I smiled to myself at the memory as I walked through the morning, at the start of the great border forests. It was so still and quiet that any noise made me turn and imagine hobbits scurrying through the trees. This was country like no other we'd come through, and so quickly had we become submerged in it I wondered what had happened to the open moors. They seemed like a long time ago.

The day turned steamy, and the gnats were out in squadrons. If you stopped for a minute they settled on you, tucked in their napkins and set to work. It was the hottest day of the trip and I was dressed in a long-sleeved shirt with my trousers tucked into my boots, walking in a miasma of sweat scented with insect repellent.

We dipped in and out of the trees, occasionally passing through areas that had been clear-cut and looked like bombsites. Huge stumps and roots had been torn up and lay on their sides lifelessly. The burnt earth around them appeared grey and contaminated. I felt I'd got here just after some disaster had struck and the dust was still settling.

It was ugly and unpleasant, and I thought: I don't want to be here; I want to be back up in the cool fells. Then I'd catch a view of the Cheviots, rising above the trees in the distance, like an island in the sea of timber. They grew each time I saw them and it became clear what the Pennine Way was up to. It had caught sight of these hills on the horizon and hadn't been able to resist them. The Cheviot range was the last challenge in England.

We emerged from the trees at last and into farmland, past more sleepy homesteads, no living thing to be seen. Mid-afternoon, and the sun was still high in the sky with another eight hours to go before its day was over. The land lay spread-eagled, pummelled senseless by the uncustomary heat. Streams were reduced to a trickle, cow-pats dried to a crisp.

Then there was the sign that any long distance walker loves to see. Nailed to a fence were the words: Refreshments at Horneystead farm, one mile. After six hours of walking through forest and moorland without so much as an ice cream van, nothing raises the spirits quite like a sign like that.

I jumped over the fence and counted the steps, imagining the farmhouse, probably a sixteenth-century stone building, wrapped in virginia creeper with rustic garden furniture to facilitate cream teas on the lawn. And there, running out to tend to the needs of passing travellers, is the lady of the house with red arms and an apron bearing a recipe for toad-in-the-hole.

We crossed the Wark's Burn, a cool stream and a shady

glade. I would have stopped and soaked my feet but there was another sign to Horneystead Farm: *This Way For Teas*, with an arrow pointing resolutely ahead. Even Boogie could understand this one. He got a sparkle in his eye, the one he only gets when he smells a cake in the oven. Now all either of us could see ahead was a table spread with chocolate sponge and flapjacks and lemon drizzle cake. My pace quickened, from walking half-heartedly with a daydream in my head I was now striding north, a rumble in my stomach.

Another sign on a fence. *This Way Teas – 100 yards*.

I'd start off with a cold drink. Then order tea for two. Then maybe have some sandwiches before the cake. Maybe I'd stay the night.

There was the farm. Not exactly sixteenth century, but old enough, a building anyway. And it had a garden, no chairs and table visible, overgrown in fact, but that was good, I liked wild gardens. No sign of any life, but the farmer's wife was probably inside putting the finishing touches to her toffee shortbread.

I walked round the house, called Hello! quietly, then loudly. Then too loudly, the cry of a desperate man.

No answer. I couldn't find a front door, so I walked round to the back. My knuckle was raised when I saw the sign in the window.

Closed Today.

I'm sure she had good reason. Maybe she'd had to take someone to hospital. Maybe she'd had to go to hospital herself. Maybe there had been a life-or-death emergency. There had better have been.

I left the farm in a dark mood which quickly descended to depression which ruined the whole day. If you're in a car and this happens you just drive onto the next place. If you're on foot, that's it, the end. No tea, no cake. The sun slips behind a cloud. The let down is

enormous. If you're walking with a dog you take it out
on him.

It took me until Bellingham to recover. I passed the
field where the agricultural show had been held on my
previous visit. Just another field, but there in the corner
was the old grandstand and I was amazed at how strong
the memory of that day was. The show had been a festival
of all things Northumbrian: bagpipes and wrestling; cattle
and pigs covered in rosettes and without a scrap of dung
on them; huge vegetables and dark fruit cakes that you
weren't allowed to eat, only look at.

I walked into the village over the River North Tyne and
looked out for the pub where I'd had such an evening, the
Fox and Hounds. But I couldn't find it, and then I realised
I was standing right outside it and it had closed down.
The sign had gone and the windows were dark. Grime
lined every frame. I peered inside. I remembered a piano
had been pushed into the hallway. Most of its keys were
stuck down with generations of beer, but we all danced
to whatever was played. Everyone drank whisky and the
farmers all wore the rosettes they'd won at the show. Now
there was no clue that this had once been a pub at all, just
the shadow on the wall where the sign used to be.

'She got too old,' said the barmaid in the Rose and
Crown referring to the woman who used to run the Fox
and Hounds. 'She retired and no-one would take it over.
It never made any money.'

Bellingham had three other pubs which all catered for
the tourists, so a place like the Fox and Hounds, that had
done no food and had damp patches on the walls, stood
little chance. I told her how I had danced and sung until
the small hours that night and she laughed and said, 'we
were all a lot younger then.'

I hadn't been that much younger then. I could still
dance and sing the night away, although the mere thought

of it now made me yawn, and my limbs begin to stiffen.

As I was leaving I smiled at the barmaid, and she said, 'Yes, it's a shame; the Fox is sadly missed. But there's nothing you can do about it, is there?'

Of course there was! Everyone in the village could have chipped in and bought the place and run it themselves. It could have been a community pub. They could have got the piano fixed and put in new seats. They could have put prints on the wall of Olde Bellingham. They could have knocked the two little bars into one big one and attracted some tourist trade if they got short of funds. They could have put fruit machines in and a telly and served pub grub with a roast Sunday dinner every day of the week. Within six months they could be overcooking their carrots. Maybe it was best left shut.

I had some fish and chips, gave Boogie a bag of batter and sat on the wall outside the shop. A blue van was parked nearby. It had familiar lines and when you looked at it closely you could see it had been converted from an old ambulance. A man was sitting on the steps polishing his spectacles. He clicked his fingers and whistled when he saw Boogie and Boogie trotted over and got a biscuit for his trouble. Boogie isn't the sort of dog to refuse treats from strangers. He'd climb in a car with any old pervert for a custard cream. The man tickled his chin and called him an old rascal, said all the things we imagine dogs like to hear but which, I suspect, makes them cringe.

I peered into his van. It was kitted out like a mobile home, but this was no tourist on a two week jolly. This man lived in here. I asked him where he was headed and he said, 'Got some friends in Bristol,' and then his story came out in a gush. He had lived happily in Lancashire but his wife had died and he had felt so depressed he went down to stay with friends in Wales. When he came back he found his house vandalised. He couldn't live there any more, so he sold up and bought this old ambulance and customised it. Now he spent his time travelling round the country, parked up in friend's gardens, two weeks here, two weeks there and the winter in Scotland.

'People think Scotland's cold in the winter, but that west coast stays nice all year round. It's the gulf stream. The fishermen up there put their hands in the sea to warm them up.'

He bought some chips and came back and sat next to me on the wall. 'I'm fortunate see,' he said. 'I've got a skill. I'm an electrician. I can fix anything. You wouldn't believe what happens when people hear I'm in the area. They come from miles around and bring me their hair dryers and electric fires.'

I could believe that. I'd love someone like that to park up outside my house. I'd throw piles of non-functional electrical goods at him. In fact if I'd known I was going to meet this man I'd have brought them along with me.

He said, 'If I was to stop here I guarantee you in a couple of days this van would be surrounded by tumble dryers.'

He was happy enough. He said he'd like to live somewhere, but he couldn't find anywhere he liked that much. He'd been wandering round for five years now and he spoke about travelling in the same way people on the Pennine Way spoke about their new found freedom: 'I just like being on the move. I like knowing when I arrive somewhere that I can always move on. And I like meeting lots of different people.'

He was hooked, and you got the feeling he said exactly the same things to everyone he met, never got beyond telling his life story. He was running from something; working something out. He'd keep going like this for a few years and then end up back in his old village in Lancashire.

The chip shop closed, the town went quiet. I phoned Catherine and told her about the man in the blue van and she said, 'Isn't it about time you got to Scotland?'

'I'm getting there.'

'Two weeks you said.'

'It's not been easy, you know. This is the Pennine Way. It's hell. In places.'

'You're not dawdling or anything, are you?'

'No.'

'Taking the long route?'

'Whatever makes you think that?'

'I've got the children to put a map up on the fridge. They've made a little red man with a pin in and they move you up every time you call in.'

'That's nice.'

'And you don't seem to be moving much.'

Maybe I was beginning to dawdle. It was difficult to stride purposefully in weather like this. The next day was even hotter than the previous. Boogie woke up panting. I smeared sun screen over myself until I glistened, then went into the village to buy a picnic. The newspapers were reporting on the heat wave now. What a Scorcher. Britain Sizzles. Drought Warning Shock. Man Walks Pennine Way and Never Gets to Wear his Waterproofs.

I certainly felt like dawdling in Bellingham. Everyone seemed to know each other's name here. Everyone was in a disgustingly good mood. Everyone patted Boogie and said good morning to me.

'I'll have some flowers for the wedding,' said Mrs Drabble in the grocer's.

'Don't forget the Summer Fayre on Saturday afternoon,' said Mr Peak in the butcher's.

'How's your neck?' asked Mavis Blake when she bumped into Angela Truscott.

'He says it could be a trapped nerve,' said poor Angela.

A man leant on his fork in his allotment, shaking his head as he examined his leeks.

'They're not growing quick enough,' he muttered when I complimented him on them, and he took his hat off and squinted accusingly at the sun.

They looked just fine to me. I watched them for a moment as if I might be able to see them growing and reassure him.

'I'm at a loss, to be honest,' he said sadly. He'd done everything he could. He'd fed them through tubes that went down deep into the soil, but they weren't performing. 'They don't stand a chance of winning.'

He was talking about the Bellingham Show, of course. His leeks needed to be cartoon parodies of themselves to get in the prizes.

'They've got to be twelve inches in circumference,' he said, and looked as though he might burst into tears. 'I think the problem is, I went and used grass-cuttings from the golf course when I should have used muck.'

I left the village reluctantly and followed the path onto the moors. The crossing of Lough Shaw heading for Whitely Pike would have been very difficult to navigate in bad conditions, but today the sky was a perfect china blue, a heat haze was rising and I even had a target to aim for. The Cheviots were in range now standing proudly on the skyline, a fortress of hills, each buttressing the other until they peaked at what was presumably the Cheviot itself. They looked like something alien that had landed on this bleak place, a worthy climax to the path. Beyond them was Scotland.

There were few villages in these wild parts, let alone towns. The border region's history was one of violent dispute, and there was never any encouragement for anyone to settle here. A system of inheritance called 'gavelkind', in which property was split between sons at the father's death, meant that over hundreds of years these parcels of land dwindled until there was hardly enough for a family to live off. Lawlessness prevailed. Theft of livestock became commonplace and, since England was richer, most of the rustlers – or reivers as they became known – came from Scotland. Marches were introduced but they had little effect. What farms there were were regularly put to the torch, and whole families butchered.

The only feature on all these moors is the bell-shaped monument on Padon Hill, a tribute to Alexander Padon. He was a Scottish Covenanter who held services up here far from authority in the seventeenth century, in the days when nonconformists, especially Scots, were persecuted. Each of his congregation was required to carry a stone up the hill to make a pile as a symbol of solidarity. The monument was built, presumably out of the original stones, in the 1920s. Boogie sniffed it and thought about cocking his leg, but desisted out of respect. I've noticed that about him over the years. He does have a degree of integrity. He will, for example, bark and growl at a postman but never one carrying registered mail.

Now the path sunk down into Redesdale Forest and began a dusty march along logging trails. You had to feel sorry for this border region really. After centuries of in-fighting it had finally settled down to a peaceful if frugal existence as a farming community, when along came a national timber shortage and it was planted with an army of conifers. Not long after that there was a water supply crisis and what land was left was drowned to build the Keilder reservoir, the biggest man-made lake in Europe.

The paths followed the fire breaks for the most part. This was dull walking but at least it provided merciful shade. These tracks were cool and sweet-smelling and, apart from the occasional logging truck which passed in a great cloud of dust, they were peaceful as could be.

Then somehow I took a wrong turning and entered the forest. Quickly I found myself submerged in this grey nether world, wandering about under the armpits of the trees where the sun never shone.

The floor was a tangle of dead wood; it was like clambering over shipwrecks. I lost any path there might have been, and when I turned round to retrace my steps, there seemed to be no way back. I headed for the one source of light I could see, which was presumably the forest edge, but this was like swimming for the shore in a rough sea, the distance much further than it seemed. I heard Boogie barking, and turned to see him stranded on a raft of logs. I went back and hauled him down, and we waded towards the edge of the forest, but there was something unnerving about all this. I came face to face with a tree with a label nailed to it: *Norway Spruce Planted 1941*. I felt locked in a cupboard with piles of potential furniture.

Eventually we emerged onto another fire break, and I sat there wet with sweat, filthy from head to foot and spitting pine needles. I felt as though I'd extricated myself from someone's grip.

We followed the path out of the trees and finally into open fields once again at Blakehopeburnhaugh, whose claim to fame is owning the longest placename in England. I spent the rest of the day trying to think of a longer one. Wasn't there a village in Suffolk called Stanburyhopetonfordwickhamdale-next-the-sea?

Byrness is the last village in England, a position confirmed by the sort of signs that gather round these outposts: *last petrol before Scotland, First Hotel in England.*

In fact it was purpose built in the 1950s, for the workers planting the forest and for the builders of the nearby

Catcleugh reservoir. As these projects were completed the houses were sold off. Now it's little more than an estate of residential dwellings on a main road, with trees grown around it forcing it into shadow.

Three of the houses have been turned into a youth hostel and this has become known as the base camp for the Cheviot traverse. The hostel warden kindly let Boogie stay. In fact I think he'd rather have had Boogie stay than me. He patted him and tickled his belly and said, 'he's champion he is,' and he gave me an extra blanket.

Four young Germans on motorbikes turned up, handsome in their leathers. They took off their helmets, let loose their long hair and then sprawled over their machines, looking dead sexy as they waited for the warden to prepare their rooms.

Later I sat with them on benches on the village green as they ate their supper in the evening sun. They said they'd motored down from Edinburgh that afternoon. I caught myself calculating how long it would take to walk to Edinburgh.

'This heat,' they said. 'There is no need for the British to go abroad for their holidays.'

I was waiting for a man to come out of the phone box, a big man who filled the little space. His voice could be heard a long way off in the still evening and I could tell he was walking the Pennine Way. He was arranging for someone to pick him up in Kirk Yetholm.

He came out and said, 'I'm very sorry to have kept you waiting. She wanted to chat.'

I recognised him now; I'd seen him the previous evening in Bellingham. I said to him, 'Are you walking the. . . ?'

'Yes I am,' he replied.

'Shall we go. . . ?'

'To the pub? Yes let's.'

We walked along the busy road. By this stage of the walk

most Pennine Walkers can finish off each other's sentences. He said to me: 'How did you cope with. . . ?'

'Black Hill? It was a morass. What did you make of. . . ?'

'Cross Fell? It was grim.'

His name was Robert and he was about fifty. He said he'd enjoyed himself thoroughly on this walk, but he'd had trouble with his feet. He looked as though he'd had trouble with his feet all his life, to be honest. His boots were worn in strange places. I imagined he got through shoes the way most people got through socks.

'Big people have a different relationship with their feet from smaller people,' he said. 'I thought I knew my feet but this trip has made me reconsider.'

The pub had burned down the previous winter but an adjacent barn had been converted into a bar, and drinkers stood there in a little corner. We bought packets of crisps, the *Win £10,000* sort. I said, 'Are you prepared for this?'

'For crisps? Yes I think so,' said Robert.

'For winning £10,000. I mean, if there is a £10,000 token in there will you still set off on the Cheviot traverse tomorrow or will you take a taxi home?'

'I live in Kent,' he said. 'Besides, to finish this walk is much more important than winning £10,000.'

Of course it was. A fifty-year-old clearing out his metaphorical attic wasn't going to be denied the Pennine Way with just one day to go. This was his moment of triumph.

We opened our crisps. Neither of us won. 'I'm not doing that again,' said Robert.

He asked me where I was going to stay the following night and I told him I hadn't decided. The Cheviot traverse was tricky because, not only was it reputed to be the most taxing section of the whole Pennine Way, it was also the longest stretch without any facilities. There were three alternatives: to press on and complete the whole, tough thirty miles in a day; to camp – although there was little shelter from the fierce winds anywhere up there; or to come down off the ridge to find accommodation in one of the valleys, although this would incur a lengthy detour and mean you would have to climb back up to the ridge the following morning.

I had planned to have a go at walking the whole thing in one day, but Robert said, 'I've noticed on the map there's a mountain hut, about twenty miles along the route. I was going to spend the night in there.'

He said it as if he was inviting me to dinner. I imagined us up there having a party on our last night on the Pennine Way, watching the moon rise over the Cheviot, recalling our exploits, how it had been tough but character building, how we had changed as human beings and had emerged as better, more tolerant people, and then we'd have a brandy and cigar each and the toast would be: The Pennines.

'Okay,' I said. I didn't fancy a thirty-mile hike in raw sunshine anyway.

'Oh well,' said Robert, downing his drink, 'Big day tomorrow, better have an early night.'

'You're right.'

'Another drink?'

'Why not.'

When he came back from the bar I said, 'You have noticed that I have a dog, haven't you?'

'Of course,' said Robert. 'Good company I bet.'

'I just point this out because there are people who might not relish the idea of spending a night in a mountain hut with Boogie. He has wind and he barks in his sleep and if you don't zip your bag up tightly he's in there in a flash.'

'He looks all right to me,' said Robert. 'He reminds me of someone. Bruce Forsyth.'

We walked back to the hostel. A cardboard sign with the words 'to Lorraine's birthday party', had been set against the fence on the side of the road. An arrow underneath pointed up a lane. I said, 'There was a time when I would have taken a sharp right here and gone and knocked on Lorraine's door and said, happy birthday Lorraine, can I come to your party?'

'You're probably old enough to be her father,' Robert said.

When we got back to the hostel I climbed up the stairs to bed, but Robert stayed in the kitchen and put some eggs on to boil. 'Just going to make some sandwiches,' he said. 'For the journey.'

When I saw him next morning he was still making egg sandwiches. A pile stood on the table like the sliced-white tower of Pisa. Food wasn't going to be a problem on this hike, that much was clear, but water might be. A month previously I'd associated the Pennine Way with wet feet and cold winds, now I was filling my pack with quart containers of water and thinking how I should ration myself, and dehydration rather than hypothermia was my worry. The day had dawned deadly hot again, and this time there'd be no shade of conifers. Up there we'd be walking across bald heads.

We had a hearty breakfast in the filling station café. The family who ran it stood there and watched us eat, saying nothing. I felt like a condemned man.

I bought some fig rolls and fruit tarts, and gave Boogie a high calorie breakfast of a packet of Jaffa Cakes. He looked at them and thought: Jaffa Cakes for Breakfast? I'm going to be put down aren't I?

Then we all set off. The last stretch, and still I felt a thrill at the thought of having nothing to do all day but walk.

And that's all today would be. There would be no diversions, no time for lingering. As the Pennine Way left Byrness it went straight up, as if to say: 'I'm not mucking about today, boys. I'm not taking prisoners. If you're only fooling, stop now and have another full breakfast in the filling station.'

We climbed slowly. Robert and I were very polite to each other. We were sounding each other out, finding what pace the other liked to walk.

'Not holding you up, am I?'

'You're not holding me up, no.'

'Go ahead if you want to.'

'No no, after you.'

'Let the dog set the pace.'

'Good idea.'

It wasn't a good idea. As soon as he reached the top of Byrness Hill, Boogie sat down.

'Dog's having a rest. Time for a little drink, I think,' said Robert.

This was disappointing since we'd only been walking twenty minutes, but encouraging in so much as Robert was making it clear early on that he wasn't a walker who liked to suffer any hardship, like a slightly dry mouth. He was a plodder, was Robert, something of which he was proud. He spoke as if he owed the position he had reached in life to his plodding. He said: 'Steady, that's me. I always get there.'

We sat down. Already the ground was simmering on this dazzling day. Boogie sat behind us, finding the only shadow on the hill. Robert already had huge sweat stains under his armpits.

'Have some of my water,' I said.

'No no,' said Robert. 'Have some of my Lemon Barley.'

We squinted at the skyline ahead. The Pennine Way

followed a complicated ridgeback through the Cheviots, complicated because there seemed to be no peaks to this range. The hills were like a nest of boils, growing out of each other.

'Egg sandwich,' said Robert, flicking an insect off the crust.

'Thank you very much.'

'Egg sandwich,' said Robert and offered one to Boogie who, as politely as he could, whipped it out of Robert's hand and swallowed in one gulp.

We pressed on. Boogie, knowing which side his bread is buttered and being a congenitally fickle little creep, now walked at Robert's side instead of mine. I walked behind, letting Robert set the pace now. He was trudging and I imagined I was doing the same. We resembled two desert rats yomping back to base after a crash landing.

But I liked Robert. He was always pulling things out of his rucsack like egg sandwiches, and boiled sweets. And he was the first walker I'd met who hadn't asked me questions about my equipment. Nor did he talk about TV sitcoms. Instead we talked about education, health, the environment and beards.

He said, 'I've been thinking of compiling a questionnaire to discover why people do this walk.'

'Why did you do it?' I got in first.

'Oh, it was something I always wanted to do.'

'And you thought you should do it now while you still could?'

'Exactly. How about you?'

'Oh, the dog needed a walk. He's suffering a midlife crisis. I thought if I took him on the Pennine Way it would rejuvenate him. Make him look like one of those dogs in the dog food commercials.'

Robert took a long look at Boogie. 'It's not really worked, has it?'

'I don't know,' I protested.

'Take my word for it,' said Robert.

'It's a difficult time for him, this realisation that he's no longer up and coming.'

'I had a midlife crisis once,' said Robert. 'I wanted to look like the man in the Gillette commercial.'

'Gillette, the best a man can get?'

'That's the one. I got myself fit, spent a lot of money on improving my appearance, spent a lot of money on Gillette toiletries. Put more energy into my career. And guess what happened?'

'What?'

'My wife left me.'

'Oh dear.'

'It was then I realised that instead of rejuvenating myself I should have indulged myself. Middle age should be embraced rather than avoided. So I decided I'd model myself on Victor Meldrew in those building society adverts. After that my wife came back and we all lived happily ever after.'

We walked in silence. It struck me I'd done this all wrong. I said, 'Are you suggesting that instead of getting back to basics on this trip, we should have been staying at the best hotels, and had a porter carry our bags?'

'Exactly,' said Robert.

'In that case, tonight we shall stay in the best accommodation available. Hear that, Boogie?'

'You mean the mountain hut,' said Robert.

'Want a fig roll?' I said.

'Good idea. 'Bout time for a little sit-down.'

We stared out over Ogre Hill. I said, 'So you never wanted this walk to change you in any way, make you a different person, fulfil any fantasies you've harboured?'

He thought about this. 'No. Although, if I'm honest, I

had hoped the regular exercise would have had a beneficial
effect on my haemorrhoids.'

'Has it?'

'No.'

These hills were so beautiful and empty, and on this
blue and green day we could see every crease in them.
The views rolled down over smooth curves into sparkling
valleys, riddled with streams. This was even wilder country
than the upper Tees, and I knew we were seeing it
under exceptional conditions. There were probably only
a handful of days like this each year. Walkers normally
spent the Cheviot traverse with the ground snapping at
their heels, trying to swallow them up, but here we were
in shorts, and the peat underfoot was soft as carpet pile.
We could have walked it in sandals.

'You know what's been the best thing for me about
The Pennine Way,' said Robert. 'The people I've met.
It's made all the difference. They've all been damn good
fellows. Even your funny-looking dog. I met one man who
spent a whole evening trying to teach me to juggle.'

And on we plodded.

There was nothing up here. The whole morning all
we passed was the empty site of a Roman Fort, a few
impressions left in the turf. When we reached the border
fence – the functional post-and-wire job that separates
Scotland from England – it was a major feature, and we
stopped and stared.

'That's some fence.'

'It's some fence all right.'

'It's well made.'

'Built to last.'

The path stuck hard to this wire as it strung a series
of ridges together, gently climbing towards the hulk
of the Cheviot. Then a hut appeared over a ridge, a
similar shelter to the one where we intended to stay

the night. Both were maintained as refuges for walkers in bad weather.

'Stop for lunch here?' suggested Robert, as if he'd just spotted a nice-looking restaurant off the A34.

Boogie slowed and in preparation opened his mouth like a letter box, just wide enough to slot an egg sandwich.

As we approached the hut I could hear giggles. Who knows what was going on inside, but it sounded a lot more fun than walking the Pennine Way. 'Hello,' I called out, the way you do, when you want to let someone know they've got ten seconds to get dressed before you come in.

The giggles stopped. Then a man emerged, blinking in the sunlight. 'Hello,' he said in a foreign accent, trying to appear to all the world like someone who hadn't come all the way from Holland to a lonely hut in the Cheviots just to fool around with his girlfriend, who was now stepping out after him.

'Lovely day,' she said.

'Lovely day,' I said.

'We are walking in the beautiful Cheviots,' she said.

'We are from Holland,' he said.

We all stood there grinning inanely as they gave us these snippets of information without provocation. The woman tucked her shirt in.

'We are as well,' I said.

The Dutchman looked surprised.

'Not Dutch,' said Robert. 'We're walking in the Cheviots.'

'It's very beautiful,' she said.

'Lovely,' I said.

'Egg sandwich,' said Robert, and he pulled one out like a rabbit from a hat.

The Dutch couple declined. Boogie ate it for them. Robert said, 'It's funny. Up here on the Cheviots in wildest England and we bump into someone from Holland.'

'Why's that funny?' asked the Dutch woman, who didn't find it funny at all.

'Don't know,' said Robert. 'Don't really know why I said it.'

The Dutch couple left, heading back to Byrness. Robert said, 'Thinking about it, everywhere you go in the world you seem to find someone from Holland.'

'I've noticed that,' I said.

The path kept to the border fence for the rest of the afternoon. We walked in silence as we grew tired from the gradients and the sun. The 2700-foot Cheviot was beginning to loom. 'Don't look at it,' said Robert. 'You'll just depress yourself.'

I was anything but depressed though. This was the finest walking of the whole trip, and The Pennine Way, as usual, followed the most dramatic, highest route.

'Well, look at that,' said Robert, pausing at a post on the fence where a grey vest hung limply. That was the full set of clothing now. I had this image of reaching Kirk Yetholm and the first thing I would see would be a naked hiker.

We climbed ever on, up Lamb Hill, down Beef Hill, Up Swinhead Hill. Then we began the steep ascent of Windy Gyle, an impressive summit at 2000 feet. I looked at Boogie and he was walking with his tongue out, but then I looked at Robert and he was as well. I hung my own tongue out in solidarity and in this fashion we reached the top.

We rested by the cairn that was piled high with stones and bleached as white as some hacienda. The view from here stretched for miles eastward to the coastal plain, and there, shimmering as it merged with the sky, was the North Sea.

'It's a mirage,' said Robert.

'No, it's the real thing.'

I looked at him. He appeared a lot older now than he had before we left that morning. He was sweating like a leaking tap, his energy draining away. As we left windy Gyle and began the climb up the flank of the Cheviot, he had to stop so frequently I began to wonder if he was all right. He was dragging his feet and starting to speak more loudly. 'And look at the bloody Health Service, it's a disgrace,' he'd yell to no-one but me.

He was overweight and worked in an office, and he was becoming flushed. I wondered what I'd do if he went and had a coronary right here in the middle of the Cheviots. I imagined having to drag him down to Kirk Yetholm, having to meet his wife and break the news. 'What were his last words?' she'd ask, and I'd lie and tell her: 'He said: "Tell my wife and children I love them,"' whereas his last words would undoubtedly be, 'just give me an egg sandwich and I'll be all right.'

We walked very slowly now. Boogie in front, all pant and froth; me second, hands over ears to stop sunburn; Robert at the rear beginning to sound like Captain Oates: 'You go on; I'm just holding you up.'

'Certainly not. We're in this together.'

Then there was a figure approaching. Such was the visibility and the terrain so bare, we could see him from a long way off, a man swinging his arms purposefully and with a pack high up his back. We took a long time to reach each other and then when we did we just stopped and stood there. We'd had twenty minutes to think of something to say and now we were too exhausted to spit out even a platitude.

Eventually he said, 'Hot isn't it?'

'I was going to say that,' I replied.

'What were you going to say?' the stranger asked Robert.

'I was going to say are you walking the . . . Pennine Way?'

The way he didn't finish Robert's sentence made it clear he wasn't. In fact he looked rather irritated that we should suggest such a thing. Instead he announced, 'I'm walking John O'Groats to Land's End actually,' and he gave us such a supercilious look that I remember thinking: smug bastard! He must have had the same effect on Robert, because he was the only person we came across that whole day to whom he didn't offer a swig of his Lemon Barley.

Now The Cheviot was in our sights. It's not the highest peak on the Pennine Way but it ought to be. It stands like an Everest, supported on all sides by failing summits. In all the pictures it's topped with cloud but today it was caught in the sun without its hat on, and it looked pale and exposed.

It wasn't actually on the path, but you could take a two-mile diversion if you wanted to reach the trig. point. We hauled ourselves up to where the path bifurcated.

'So, are we going to climb the peak of The Cheviot?' I asked with as much enthusiasm as I could manage.

Robert looked at the trail heading up up up to the right. 'No,' he said, and he turned down down down to the left.

Don't look at me, intimated Boogie and followed Robert down.

'I guess not then,' I said and followed them both.

Then the second mountain refuge hut, our shelter for the night, came in view. It was almost eight o'clock by now and I was glad that this was as far as we were going. My ears were burning and knees trembling, and we descended down the steep slope with thoughts of warm soup and cold beer and feather down mattresses, which was stupid when all we had was egg sandwiches and jam tarts, and a floor to crash on.

To our right the Hen Hole appeared, a deep gash in these otherwise smooth-sided hills, looking like an open mouth with a sore throat, and falling fast into shadow.

Beyond that The Schill rose, the first climb of the following morning and the last climb of the whole walk. From there the land dropped gently away and somewhere below was Kirk Yetholm.

We trudged up to the refuge hut door. 'After you,' I said to Robert.

'No no, after you, I insist,' he replied. He was suffering from sun stroke, dehydration, exhaustion and sore feet, but he didn't let this affect his manners.

I pushed open the door and stumbled in, and there were three other hikers sitting on a bench against the wall.

'Evening,' said one.

'Evening,' I said.

'Good evening,' said Robert.

'Are you walking the . . . ?' they said

'Yes we are. . . .' I replied

'So are we.'

We introduced ourselves. Two of them, Ray and Mike, were in their sixties and walking together. The other, Bernie, was thirty-something and on his own. They looked beaten by the sun. Bernie's nose was in a bad way. Ray was shivering with sun stroke. It didn't matter what conditions were like on these hills, if you were out in them all day they drained you one way or another.

I asked, 'Are you staying here the. . . ?'

'Night? Yes we are,' said Ray. 'Are you staying. . . ?'

I looked round. A hut was a good description for this place. It was four wooden walls with a little window and a roof and this bench.

'If that's all right with you gentlemen?' asked Robert.

'Fine with us,' said Ray.

They shuffled up to make room on the bench and Boogie jumped and stretched out, taking up three places.

'Has that dog walked the Pennine Way?' asked Mike.

'Yes,' I said and noted pride in my voice.

'Give him a biscuit, Ray.'

Ray dug in his bag and pulled out a biscuit. Boogie swallowed it whole with a '271 miles I've walked! It's worth a packet of these.'

'Would anyone like an egg sandwich?' asked Robert.

He pulled out a crumpled plastic bag that contained a few crumbs and yellow pebbles of egg. 'Oh,' he said.

Our new friends were better equipped. 'There's no worry about food,' said Bernie. 'We've got loads; it's our last night, we're going to eat everything in our rucsacks.'

'Except Ray's laundry,' said Mike.

'We can have a feast,' said Bernie.

They emptied their bags of provisions and gathered together tins of corned beef and baked beans, a packet of Cadbury's Smash, some pickled onions, crackers, some Marmite. . . .

'See,' said Bernie, 'a feast.'

'Anyone mind if I take my boots off?' asked Robert.

'Make yourself at home,' said Ray.

'I can contribute some individual fruit pies,' I said, 'and some complete dog food.'

'The pies sound nice,' said Bernie.

'What sort of dog food did you say it was?' asked Mike.

'Complete.'

'I've never tried that,' he said.

I pulled out the box of fruit pies I'd bought in Byrness. They were nothing but sticky crumbs.

'Lovely,' said Mike.

'The question is,' said Ray, 'what shall we cook?'

'I want this last meal to be memorable,' said Mike.

'A Pennine Way special I think,' said Bernie.

'You mean put everything in a frying pan and make a hash of it?' suggested Ray.

'Exactly,' said Bernie.

'You could put some marmite in it for a sauce,' said Mike.

'Grand idea,' said Ray.

'Yes, grand idea,' said Robert, who had got his boots off and was now looking inside them for any missing parts of his feet.

The hut filled with a Marmite-scented fug. We brewed some tea and sat there warming our hands on mugs as a wind picked up outside.

'Glad I'm not in a tent tonight,' said Mike. 'There's something blowing in.'

The meal was quickly ready. It was a mush of corned beef and baked beans, Cadbury's Smash, pickled onions and Marmite sauce. It was the best meal I'd had on the Pennine Way.

The scrape of plates and the sound of the wind. Five Pennine Way walkers with suntanned heads and baggy eyes, on their last night. Ray licked his plate and belched. 'Well that filled the gap.'

'My compliments to the chef,' said Robert, and licked his fingers.

A chill blew round the hut. We all climbed into our sleeping bags and lay around the floor waiting for it to get dark. Boogie farted but nobody minded. There was a team spirit in that hut that night that mere flatulence couldn't undermine.

I said, 'I don't like to say it, but I've been very disappointed by the Pennine Way.'

'Why's that?' asked Ray.

'I set out expecting it to be a mindless trudge through fog and bog, that would do little but make me appreciate what I'd left behind. But it hasn't been like that at all. In fact I have to confess I didn't find Black Hill to be a morass. I found it to be very interesting and beautiful in a peaty sort of way. The same with Bleaklow. And I've decided I'd like my ashes to be scattered over Swaledale.'

'That's understandable,' said Ray.

Then Bernie said, 'To be honest, I'm disappointed in it as well. I came thinking it was the place I'd be least likely to meet a woman. And then I go and fall for the daughter of the camp site owner in Hebden Bridge.'

'Very attractive she was,' said Ray.

'I've spent most of this trip dreaming that one day we'll get married at Tan Hill Inn.'

'I'll be your best man,' said Ray.

And Mike said, 'I've loved every minute. I've been so impressed with the Pennine Way, I've penned a thirty-five verse poem in rhyming couplets singing its praises. Would you like to hear it?'

'No, we bloody wouldn't,' said Ray who had heard it every night since The Bowes Gap.

Robert said, 'This walk has inspired me to the extent that I'm thinking of standing for parliament in the next election as the Independent member for Bromsgrove.'

'I'll vote for you,' said Ray.

There was an end-of-term feeling. Mike and Ray were retired and were going home to their gardens. Bernie had to go back to work in two days' time, but he said, 'I'm looking forward to seeing their faces in the office. They never believed I could do it.'

Robert mused, 'Was there ever a moment when you felt like packing up?'

We all thought about this and Ray confessed, 'There was

once, when I discovered I was beginning to find sheep attractive.'

There was a silence until I admitted, 'Actually, there was a point where I began to find sheep attractive too.'

'And me,' said Robert. 'I'll never forget a certain little Swaledale I met near Malham Tarn.'

'That's weird that is,' said Mike.

'It is,' said Bernie; 'South Country Cheviot are much prettier.'

'The Scotch Blackface have nicer legs,' said Ray.

'I rather like them petite like the Derbyshire Gritstone breed,' said Robert.

We all lay there dreaming of encounters we'd had with attractive sheep. Mike said, 'Do you think this says something strange about us?'

'There's nothing strange about finding animals attractive,' said Robert, trying to be supportive.

'It's probably very natural – on a walk of this nature,' I said.

'Exactly,' said Ray. 'To be honest I find your dog quite attractive.'

'So do I,' said Bernie.

'Me too,' said Robert. 'Now I've got to know him.'

Boogie edged further into the corner of the room, but he had no need to worry, we were all very tired. We slowly lapsed into silence. After a while I said, 'I've walked the Pennine Way and not got wet once,' but everyone was asleep.

I woke at first light as the window started to rattle. Cloud had smothered the hut like a pillow over a face, and the wind was racing down the valley from The Cheviot. I stuck my head out of the door and was hit by an icy blast.

I hurriedly dressed. The cloud looked full of rain and I wanted to get moving while there was still a bit of visibility.

I packed up and said goodbye to anyone who was awake, then stepped outside. Boogie staggered alongside me with bleary eyes and a 'what the . . . ?' expression. It was five o'clock.

Within half a mile the cloud had covered all the hills. The hut had vanished and the rain started to pour. I put my waterproofs on and Boogie barked nervously at the strange red thing now walking alongside him.

I followed the path up The Schill, visibility down to twenty metres now. It was like walking inside a bottle of smoke. I only knew I was heading uphill because of the sensation in my legs, and I could tell when I had got to the top of The Schill as the wind and rain lashed me, trying to wipe the smile off my face, but I was loving this.

'It's raining, Boogie!' I screamed above the gale. 'It's pouring!' He was standing right next to me using me as a windbreak and an umbrella.

Within minutes the rain had pierced my waterproofs. Trickles slipped down my neck and through the zip. The dry puddles on the ground filled and soon I was surrounded by bog. I splashed through it all gleefully, until one puddle gave way and I went up to my knee.

Shortly after that I lost the path in the mist. I wandered round splashing through mud for a bit then I took my compass out and discovered I was veering off towards Wales rather than Scotland.

I turned to retrace my steps, then slipped and fell on my face and turned my ankle. Water got into my boot and somewhere I lost my Swiss Army knife. As we finally climbed the stile over the fence that is the border, and set foot into Scotland, my map blew out of my hands and I never saw it again. It had been raining for an hour and I had gone from euphoria at being finally accepted by the elements, to being totally fed up with the Pennine Way and with walking in general. I was beginning to feel as depressed as a Yorkshire sheep farmer, yelling things like: 'bloody weather!' and 'typical, isn't it? You come out for a walk and look what happens.' If there had been a Pennine Way walkers' logbook nailed to a post here I would have written in it: 'Absolute misery; this is hell; Rain rain rain, that's the Pennine Way for you!'

I talked to Boogie to try to keep spirits up, but he wasn't interested, so I talked to myself:

'Where did you get those waterproofs from?' I asked.

'Hill and Dale near Sheffield,' I replied.

'Oh yeah. How much were they?' I asked.

'Thirty-six quid the set,' I replied.

'Not Gore-tex then?' I said.

'No, they're made from newspaper,' I said.

'Any good?' I asked.

'Complete crap,' I replied.

'Where did you get your boots?' I inquired.

'Oh, I took them off the feet of a dead walker I found on Black Hill.'

At last the path began to wind down, out of the hills into the lowlands. Visibility began to improve. The rain reduced to a drizzle. A dwelling came into view and then we were following a metalled track. I looked back once and saw the hills disappear into the weather.

Now I could hear a church clock chiming from over a ridge. We climbed one last hill and there in the valley below was a scattering of houses that could only be Kirk Yetholm.

I slowed and walked quietly into the village, past windows with curtains still drawn, folk sleeping-in on this Saturday morning. Then we were stepping onto the green outside the village pub, and I came to a halt in the middle, and stood there dripping, wondering what I was supposed to do now.

It was a strangely anti-climactic end. But what had I

been expecting? A fanfare, with the parish council lining the road to applaud me in? I sat on a bench, hoping a human being might appear and slap me on the back and say well done. But when someone did walk past they didn't lift their head from their newspaper. I was just another wet and muddy bloke who had walked into town.

I had to speak to someone. I phoned home. I wanted to tell them we'd done it. I wanted to say, get the champagne on ice.

The answer-machine clicked on – it was seven o'clock in the morning. I listened to my own voice, then left a message, we'd be home that night.

Outside the box I turned to Boogie and said, 'Boogie, congratulations! You have completed the Pennine Way.'

His face could possibly have said: congratulations to you as well. But more than likely said: so how come the pub isn't open?

I fed him breakfast, the last of his complete dog food. There was that damned complete dog, still bounding across the front of the packet. There was no use pretending, Boogie looked nothing like him. I screwed up the packet and threw it in a bin. I said to him, 'Do you want the good news or the bad news? The bad news. Right. The bad news is that even after 276 miles of sweat and toil and getting back to basics, you still don't look anything like the complete dog.'

'The good news, however, is that it's not important. Midlife, I've discovered, is like a bridge between youth and age. And, all credit to you, instead of resisting the crossing as most males do, you've taken it in your stride. It appears you are a perfectly well-adjusted, middle-aged dog.'

And he gave me a look that was like: well now you've got that out of your system, maybe if we hurry we could get home in time to catch the end of Wimbledon.

Getting out of Kirk Yetholm wasn't going to be so straightforward, though. The easiest option could well have been to walk the Pennine Way back home. I peered round looking for some life, but this place was like an empty filmset.

Then a man wearing waterproofs and carrying a pack on his back strolled across the green, came over when he saw me. He looked very excited. It was obvious that he was about to start what, it was equally obvious, I had just completed.

'Did you enjoy it?' he asked eagerly.

'It's magnificent,' I said. 'Spectacular. It's the best walk you'll ever do.'

His eyes sparkled: 'I've been wanting to do it for years. It's always been an ambition of mine. I thought I'd better do it while I still can. I want to . . . to. . . .'

'Find the man within?'

He blushed. 'Yeah. Sort of.'

'Prove to yourself you've still got what it takes; show them back at the office that you're still in your prime, that you can hack it with the youngsters. Improve your appearance and increase your longevity.'

'Well. . . .'

'In which case my advice is, pack up now and go and take a fortnight's package holiday to Skiathos.'

'Huh.'

'Huh.'

'You're just saying that.'

'Yeah. You'll be fine. One thing you should know though. The Pennine Way doesn't cure haemorrhoids.'

'I'll remember that.'

'And the good news is, it doesn't rain on the Pennine Way. The bad weather is just down here. Once you're up in the hills it's like flying, you're above the clouds. Hope you've got a bottle of factor 10 with you.'

We shook hands and he headed out. I strolled round Kirk Yetholm. For three weeks this place had been my destination and I wanted it to make an impression upon me. I glanced in a couple of rubbish bins; I peered in a couple of living rooms; just an unfamiliar, hairy and weathered face that peered back at me. Then in the reflection I saw two people with backpacks walking across the square. They were waving. I turned and saw Doug and Tony from Liverpool. I felt so pleased to see them.

Tony said, 'I said to Doug, that's that bloke who's not walking the Pennine Way.'

'Didn't recognise you, to be honest,' said Doug. 'You look different.'

'So do you,' I said. 'You look very well.'

'You look wet and dirty,' said Tony.

'Thank you very much,' I said.

We congratulated each other on completing the path. Doug patted Boogie and said, 'I bet this one wants to walk back as well.' It was the first time since leaving home that I heard Boogie growl in anger.

'There's our bus, look,' Doug said. 'Are you coming?'

A bus had pulled up and I thought, rather like a train on the Settle-Carlisle line, if a bus comes while you're in Kirk Yetholm, it's probably a good idea to get on it no matter where it's going.

We climbed on board. The bus was full of shoppers going into Kelso. The doors hissed shut and Doug asked, 'Did you see that bloke in the front seat?'

'What about him?' said Tony.

'He was wearing Paramo trousers. You know, those temperature-controlled ones.'

'Get away.'

Doug and Tony found seats in the back and discussed trousers. I sat over a wheel next to a woman in a pink tracksuit. 'Sorry,' I said to her.'I'm wet and muddy.'

'So's your dog. Where have you had him?'

'He's just walked the Pennine Way.'

'No wonder he looks fed up.'

'Three weeks of walking. He ate fifteen kilos of reconstituted dog food. . . .'

'Tch. Poor thing. I think I've got a paracetamol in my bag.'

'. . . .while I ate a record number of fried eggs, a fridge freezer full of cod in batter, twenty-one sticky puddings and ten pounds of carrots mashed into a mush.'

'I've got some chocolate fingers here as well, I think. . . .'

And so Boogie munched on chocolate fingers all the way to Kelso, happy to be putting on calories again. I sat there, listening to the Scottish accents all around me, already feeling as though the Pennine Way had happened to someone else. Before I left I'd had this fantasy that being out of the house for three weeks would change me beyond recognition. My family would open the door to this dark and moody stranger, an unpredictable, unsettled man who would never be able to live at home contentedly again after the terrible and wonderful things he had seen on his travels in the Pennines. He'd be prone to long silences and periods when he just wanted to be with sheep. But now, sitting here in the warm, what I felt was a wonderfully satisfying sense of normality, as if I'd fallen back to earth and landed right here in the luxury of this bus, wet and smelly, with dog hairs stuck to my clothes, steam rising off me and the engine humming me to sleep.

Also by Mark Wallington . . .

TRAVELS WITH BOOGIE

Five Hundred Mile Walkies and *Boogie Up the River* — now in one volume

Travels With Boogie is the story of two city slickers – one an unattractive but streetwise mongrel from Stockwell, the other the long-suffering author – and how they came to terms with England's countryside and waterways.

First they had to survive against all odds as they embarked on a heroic journey up hill and down dale, with rucksacks full of Kennomeat, along Britain's longest coastal footpath – from Somerset to Devon, from Cornwall to Dorset. And they did it. Then, undaunted, they took on the treacherous waters of the Thames. Not exactly as Mark had planned, however: this time his companion was to be the delectable Jennifer – but she was held up at the office, and when Boogie was dropped off at the kennels the other dogs complained.

Travels With Boogie is a witty and fascinating account of a mismatched couple and of the people they meet and the places they visit.

'Splendid reading . . . "I liked the serendipitous quality of travelling unbriefed," said the script- and travel-writer Wallington, and you certainly will too, as page after page of the south-west landscape unfolds' *Liverpool Daily Post*

'The humorous travel book we've been waiting for'
Daily Mail

Also in Arrow . . .

MOSCOW MULE

James Young

'An English version of P.J. O'Rourke' David Sinclair,
The Times

In 1993 James Young began a series of journeys to post-Glasnost Russia, uncovering a cockroach-plagued society on the verge of a vodka-fuelled nervous breakdown. The result is a masterpiece of satire, holding a looking glass up to a continent of growing tribalism emerging from the cracks of the collapsed Soviet system. Sparkling with wit and observation, with an array of eccentric characters, *Moscow Mule* puts James Young firmly in the tradition of Bill Bryson and Paul Theroux.

'Magical . . . it would be hilarious were it not all so very sad'
Tom Hibbert, *Mail on Sunday*

'Quite possibly the most perceptive and distinctive travel book of the year – Young could evolve into a travel writer of the class of Theroux and Morris' Mick Middles,
Manchester Evening News

OTHER TITLES AVAILABLE

☐ Travels With Boogie	Mark Wallington	£ 5.99
☐ Moscow Mule	James Young	£ 6.99
☐ Ice Fall in Norway	Ranulph Fiennes	£ 5.99
☐ Mind Over Matter	Ranulph Fiennes	£ 5.99
☐ To the Ends of the Earth	Ranulph Fiennes	£ 5.99
☐ The Good Guide to the Lakes	Hunter Davies	£ 5.99
☐ Running With the Moon	Jonny Bealby	£ 7.99

ALL ARROW BOOKS ARE AVAILABLE THROUGH MAIL ORDER OR FROM YOUR LOCAL BOOKSHOP.

PAYMENT MAY BE MADE USING ACCESS, VISA, MASTER-CARD, DINERS CLUB, SWITCH AND AMEX, OR CHEQUE, EUROCHEQUE AND POSTAL ORDER (STERLING ONLY).

EXPIRY DATE .... SWITCH ISSUE NO.

SIGNATURE ....

PLEASE ALLOW £2.50 FOR POST AND PACKING FOR THE FIRST BOOK AND £1.00 PER BOOK THEREAFTER.

ORDER TOTAL: £................................ (INCLUDING P&P)

ALL ORDERS TO:
ARROW BOOKS, BOOKS BY POST, TBS LIMITED, THE BOOK SERVICE, COLCHESTER ROAD, FRATING GREEN, COLCHESTER, ESSEX, CO7 7 DW, UK.

TELEPHONE: (01206) 256 000
FAX: (01206) 255 914

NAME ....

ADDRESS...

....

Please allow 28 days for delivery. Please tick box if you do not wish to receive any additional information. ☐
Prices and availability subject to change without notice.